IARC MONOGRAPHS

ON THE

EVALUATION OF THE CARCINOGENIC RISK

OF CHEMICALS TO MAN:

Some Miscellaneous Pharmaceutical Substances

Volume 13

This publication represents the views of an
IARC Working Group on the
Evaluation of the Carcinogenic Risk of Chemicals to Man
which met in Lyon,
18-25 October 1976

IARC WORKING GROUP ON THE EVALUATION OF THE CARCINOGENIC RISK OF CHEMICALS
TO MAN: SOME MISCELLANEOUS PHARMACEUTICAL SUBSTANCES

Lyon, 18-25 October 1976

Members[1]

Dr L. Bahna, Head, Department of Chemical Carcinogenesis, Cancer Research
    Institute, Slovak Academy of Sciences, ul. Cs. armady 21,
    880 32 Bratislava, Czechoslovakia

Professor L. Fiore-Donati, Director, Istituto di Anatomia e Istologia
    Patologica, Policlinico Borgo Roma, 37100 Verona, Italy

Dr P. Grasso, Deputy Director and Chief Pathologist, The British Industrial
    Biological Research Association (BIBRA), Woodmansterne Road, Carshalton,
    Surrey SM5 4DS, UK

Dr T. Hirayama, Chief, Epidemiology Division, National Cancer Center Research
    Institute, Tsukiji 5-chome, Chuo-ku, Tokyo, Japan

Professor D.B. Ludlum, Albany Medical College, Department of Pharmacology
    and Experimental Therapeutics, Albany, New York 12208, USA

Dr L. Massé, Ecole Nationale de la Santé Publique, 35043 Rennes Cédex,
    France (Vice-Chairman)

Dr J. McCann, Department of Biochemistry, University of California, Berkeley,
    California 94720, USA

Dr V.B. Okulov, N. Petrov Research Institute of Oncology, Leningradskaya
    Street 68, Pesochny-2, Leningrad 188646, USSR

Professor R. Preussmann, Deutsches Krebsforschungszentrum, Institut für
    Toxikologie und Chemotherapie, Im Neuenheimer Feld 280, Postfach 101949,
    6900 Heidelberg 1, FRG (Chairman)

Professor A. Somogyi, Bundesgesundheitsamt, Thiclallee 88/92, Postfach -
    1000 Berlin 33, FRG

Dr G.M. Williams, Chief, Division of Experimental Pathology, Naylor Dana
    Institute for Disease Prevention, American Health Foundation, Valhalla,
    New York 10595, USA

---

[1]Unable to attend: Professor D.B. Clayson, Deputy Director, The Eppley
Institute for Research in Cancer, University of Nebraska Medical Center,
42nd and Dewey Avenue, Omaha, Nebraska 68105, USA; Professor S. Garattini,
Director, Istituto di Ricerche Farmacologiche "Mario Negri", Via Eritrea 62,
20157 Milan, Italy

Invited Guest

Dr K.E. McCaleb, Director, Chemical-Environmental Program, Chemical Industries Center, Stanford Research Institute, Menlo Park, California 94025, USA (*Rapporteur sections 2.1 and 2.2*)

Representative from the National Cancer Institute

Dr S. Siegel, Coordinator, Technical Information Activities, Bioassay and Carcinogenesis Program, Division of Cancer Cause and Prevention, National Cancer Institute, Bethesda, Maryland 20014, USA

Secretariat

Dr C. Agthe, Chief, Food Additives Unit, WHO, Geneva

Dr H. Bartsch, Unit of Chemical Carcinogenesis (*Rapporteur section 3.2*)

Dr J.F. Bertaux, Medical Officer, Pharmaceuticals, WHO, Geneva

Dr A. Davis, Chief, Schistosomiasis and Other Helminthic Infections, WHO, Geneva

Dr L. Griciute, Chief, Unit of Environmental Carcinogens

Mrs D. Mietton, Unit of Chemical Carcinogenesis (*Library Assistant*)

Dr R. Montesano, Unit of Chemical Carcinogenesis (*Rapporteur section 3.1*)

Mrs C. Partensky, Unit of Chemical Carcinogenesis (*Technical editor*)

Mrs I. Peterschmitt, Unit of Chemical Carcinogenesis, WHO, Geneva (*Bibliographic researcher*)

Dr V. Ponomarkov, Unit of Chemical Carcinogenesis

Dr R. Saracci, Unit of Epidemiology and Biostatistics (*Rapporteur section 3.3*)

Dr L. Tomatis, Chief, Unit of Chemical Carcinogenesis (*Head of the Programme and Secretary*)

Mr E.A. Walker, Unit of Environmental Carcinogens (*Rapporteur sections 1 and 2.3*)

Mrs E. Ward, Montignac, France (*Editor*)

Mr J.D. Wilbourn, Unit of Chemical Carcinogenesis (*Co-secretary*)

Note to the reader

Every effort is made to present the monographs as accurately as possible without unduly delaying their publication. Nevertheless, mistakes have occurred and are still likely to occur. In the interest of all users of these monographs, readers are requested to communicate any errors observed to the Unit of Chemical Carcinogenesis of the International Agency for Research on Cancer, Lyon, France, in order that these can be included in corrigenda which will appear in subsequent volumes.

Since the monographs are not intended to be a review of the literature and contain only data considered relevant by the Working Group, it is not possible for the reader to determine whether a certain study was considered or not. However, research workers who are aware of important published data that may change the evaluation are requested to make them available to the above-mentioned address, in order that they can be considered for a possible re-evaluation by a future Working Group.

CONTENTS

BACKGROUND AND PURPOSE OF THE IARC PROGRAMME ON THE EVALUATION
OF THE CARCINOGENIC RISK OF CHEMICALS TO MAN 9

SCOPE OF THE MONOGRAPHS 9

MECHANISM FOR PRODUCING THE MONOGRAPHS 10

GENERAL PRINCIPLES FOR THE EVALUATION 11

EXPLANATORY NOTES ON THE MONOGRAPHS 14

GENERAL REMARKS ON THE SUBSTANCES CONSIDERED 23

THE MONOGRAPHS

    Acriflavinium chloride 31

    Aurothioglucose 39

    Chloroquine 47

    Diazepam and oxazepam 57

    Dithranol 75

    Ethionamide 83

    Hycanthone and hycanthone mesylate 91

    8-Hydroxyquinoline 101

    Metronidazole 113

    Niridazole 123

    Oxymetholone 131

    Phenacetin 141

    Phenobarbital and phenobarbital sodium 157

    Phenylbutazone and oxyphenbutazone 183

    Phenytoin and phenytoin sodium 201

    Pronetalol hydrochloride 227

    Pyrimethamine 233

SUPPLEMENTARY CORRIGENDA TO VOLUMES 1-12 243

CUMULATIVE INDEX TO MONOGRAPHS 245

BACKGROUND AND PURPOSE OF THE IARC PROGRAMME ON THE EVALUATION OF THE CARCINOGENIC RISK OF CHEMICALS TO MAN

The International Agency for Research on Cancer (IARC) initiated in 1971 a programme to evaluate the carcinogenic risk of chemicals to man. This programme was supported by a Resolution of the Governing Council at its Ninth Session concerning the role of IARC in providing government authorities with expert, independent scientific opinion on environmental carcinogenesis.

In view of the importance of the project and in order to expedite production of monographs, the National Cancer Institute of the United States has provided IARC with additional funds for this purpose.

The objective of the programme is to elaborate and publish in the form of monographs critical reviews of carcinogenicity and related data in the light of the present state of knowledge, with the final aim of evaluating the data in terms of possible human risk, and at the same time to indicate where additional research efforts are needed.

SCOPE OF THE MONOGRAPHS

The monographs summarize the evidence for the carcinogenicity of individual chemicals and other relevant information on the basis of data compiled, reviewed and evaluated by a Working Group of experts. No recommendations are given concerning preventive measures or legislation, since these matters depend on risk-benefit evaluations, which seem best made by individual governments and/or international agencies such as WHO and ILO.

Since 1971, when the programme was started, twelve volumes have been published[1-12]. As new data on chemicals for which monographs have already been prepared and new principles for evaluation become available, re-evaluations will be made at future meetings, and revised monographs will be published as necessary.

The monographs are distributed to international and governmental agencies, are available to industries and scientists dealing with these chemicals and are offered to any interested reader through their world-wide distribution as a WHO publication. They also form the basis of advice from IARC on carcinogenesis from these substances.

MECHANISM FOR PRODUCING THE MONOGRAPHS

As a first step, a list of chemicals for possible consideration by the Working Group is established. IARC then collects pertinent references regarding physico-chemical characteristics*, production and use*, occurrence* and analysis* and biological data** on these compounds. The material on biological aspects is summarized by an expert consultant or an IARC staff member, who prepares the first draft, which in some cases is sent to another expert for comments. The drafts are circulated to all members of the Working Group about one month before the meeting. During the meeting, further additions to and deletions from the data are agreed upon, and a final version of comments and evaluation on each compound is adopted.

Priority for the preparation of monographs

Priority is given mainly to chemicals belonging to particular chemical groups and for which there is at least some suggestion of carcinogenicity from observations in animals and/or man and evidence of human exposure. However, *the inclusion of a particular compound in a volume does not necessarily mean that it is considered to be carcinogenic. Equally, the fact that a substance has not yet been considered does not imply that it is without carcinogenic hazard.*

Data on which the evaluation is based

With regard to the biological data, only published articles and papers already accepted for publication are reviewed. The monographs are not intended to be a full review of the literature, and they contain only data considered relevant by the Working Group. Research workers who are aware

---

*Data provided by Chemical Industries Center, Stanford Research Institute, Menlo Park, California, USA

**In the collection of original data reference was made to the series of publications 'Survey of Compounds which have been Tested for Carcinogenic Activity'[13-18]. Most information on mutagenicity was provided by The Environmental Mutagen Information Center, Oakridge, Tenn., USA.

of important data (published or accepted for publication) that may influence the evaluation are invited to make them available to the Unit of Chemical Carcinogenesis of the International Agency for Research on Cancer, Lyon, France.

The Working Group

The tasks of the Working Group are five-fold: (1) to ascertain that all data have been collected; (2) to select the data relevant for the evaluation; (3) to determine whether the data, as summarized, will enable the reader to follow the reasoning of the committee; (4) to judge the significance of results of experimental and epidemiological studies; and (5) to make an evaluation of carcinogenicity.

The members of the Working Group who participated in the consideration of particular substances are listed at the beginning of each publication. The members serve in their individual capacities as scientists and not as representatives of their governments or of any organization with which they are affiliated.

GENERAL PRINCIPLES FOR THE EVALUATION

The general principles for evaluation of carcinogenicity were elaborated by previous Working Groups and also applied to the substances covered in this volume.

Terminology

The term 'chemical carcinogenesis' in its widely accepted sense is used to indicate the induction or enhancement of neoplasia by chemicals. It is recognized that, in the strict etymological sense, this term means the induction of cancer; however, common usage has led to its employment to denote the induction of various types of neoplasms. The terms 'tumourigen', 'oncogen' and 'blastomogen' have all been used synonymously with 'carcinogen', although occasionally 'tumourigen' has been used specifically to denote the induction of benign tumours.

Response to carcinogens

In general, no distinction is made between the induction of tumours and the enhancement of tumour incidence, although it is noted that there may be fundamental differences in mechanisms that will eventually be elucidated. The response of experimental animals to a carcinogen may take several forms: a significant increase in the incidence of one or more of the same types of neoplasms as found in control animals; the occurrence of types of neoplasms not observed in control animals; and/or a decreased latent period for the production of neoplasms as compared with that in control animals.

Purity of the compounds tested

In any evaluation of biological data with respect to a possible carcinogenic risk, particular attention must be paid to the purity of the chemicals tested and to their stability under conditions of storage or administration. Information on purity and stability is given, when available, in the monographs.

Qualitative aspects

In many instances, both benign and malignant tumours are induced by chemical carcinogens. There are so far few recorded instances in which only benign tumours are induced by chemicals that have been studied extensively. Their occurrence in experimental systems has been taken to indicate the possibility of an increased risk of malignant tumours also.

In experimental carcinogenesis, the type of cancer seen may be the same as that recorded in human studies, e.g., bladder cancer in man, monkeys, dogs and hamsters after administration of 2-naphthylamine. In other instances, however, a chemical may induce other types of neoplasms at different sites in various species, e.g., benzidine induces hepatic carcinoma in rats but bladder carcinoma in man.

Quantitative aspects

Dose-response studies are important in the evaluation of human and animal carcinogenesis: the confidence with which a carcinogenic effect can be established is strengthened by the observation of an increasing incidence of neoplasms with increasing exposure. In addition, such studies form the only basis on which a minimal effective dose can be established, allowing some comparison with data for human exposure.

Comparison of compounds with regard to potency can only be made when the substances have been tested simultaneously.

Animal data in relation to the evaluation of risk to man

At the present time no attempt can be made to interpret the animal data directly in terms of human risk, since no objective criteria are available to do so. The critical assessments of the validity of the animal data given in these monographs are intended to assist national and/or international authorities in making decisions concerning preventive measures or legislation. In this connection attention is drawn to WHO recommendations in relation to food additives[19], drugs[20] and occupational carcinogens[21].

Evidence of human carcinogenicity

Evaluation of the carcinogenic risk to man of suspected environmental agents rests on purely observational studies. Such studies must cover a sufficient variation in levels of human exposure to allow a meaningful relationship between cancer incidence and exposure to a given chemical to be established. Difficulties arise in isolating the effects of individual agents, however, since people are usually exposed to multiple carcinogens.

The initial suggestion of a relationship between an agent and disease often comes from case reports of patients with similar exposures. Variations and time trends in regional or national cancer incidences, or their correlation with regional or national 'exposure' levels, may also provide valuable insights. Such observations by themselves cannot, however, in most circumstances be regarded as conclusive evidence of carcinogenicity.

The most satisfactory epidemiological method is to compare the cancer risk (adjusted for age, sex and other confounding variables) among groups or cohorts, or among individuals exposed to various levels of the agent in question, and among control groups not so exposed. Ideally, this is accomplished directly, by following such groups forward in time (prospectively) to determine time relationships, dose-response relationships and other aspects of cancer induction. Large cohorts and long observation periods are required to provide sufficient cases for a statistically valid comparison.

An alternative to prospective investigation is to assemble cohorts from past records and to evaluate their subsequent morbidity or mortality by means of medical histories and death certificates. Such occupational carcinogens as nickel, β-naphthylamine, asbestos and benzidine have been confirmed by this method. Another method is to compare the past exposures of a defined group of cancer cases with those of control samples from the hospital or general population. This does not provide an absolute measure of carcinogenic risk but can indicate the relative risks associated with different levels of exposure. Indirect means (e.g., interviews or tissue residues) of measuring exposures which may have commenced many years before can constitute a major source of error. Nevertheless, such 'case-control' studies can often isolate one factor from several suspected agents and can thus indicate which substance should be followed up by cohort studies.

EXPLANATORY NOTES ON THE MONOGRAPHS

In sections 1, 2 and 3 of each monograph, except for minor remarks, the data are recorded as given by the author, whereas the comments by the Working Group are given in section 4, headed 'Comments on Data Reported and Evaluation'.

Chemical and Physical Data (section 1)

The Chemical Abstracts Registry Serial Number and the latest Chemical Abstracts Name are recorded in this section. Other synonyms and trade names are given, but this list is not intended to be comprehensive. It should also be noted that some of the trade names are those of mixtures in which the compound being evaluated is only one of the active ingredients.

Chemical and physical properties include, in particular, data that might be relevant to carcinogenicity (for example, lipid solubility) and those that concern identification. All chemical data in this section refer to the pure substance, unless otherwise specified.

Production, Use, Occurrence and Analysis (section 2)

The purpose of this section is to indicate the extent of possible human exposure. With regard to data on production, use and occurrence, IARC has collaborated with the Stanford Research Institute, USA, with the support of the National Cancer Institute of the USA. Since cancer is a delayed toxic effect, past use and production data are also provided.

The United States, Europe and Japan are reasonably representative industrialized areas of the world, and if data on production or use are available from these countries they are reported. It should *not*, however, be inferred that these nations are the sole or even the major sources of any individual chemical.

Production data are obtained from both governmental and trade publications in the three geographic areas. In some cases, separate production data on chemicals manufactured in the US were not available, for proprietary reasons. However, the fact that a manufacturer acknowledges production of a chemical to the US International Trade Commission implies that annual production of that chemical is greater than 450 kg or that its annual sales exceed $1000. Information on use and occurrence is obtained by a review of published data, complemented by direct contact with manufacturers of the chemical in question; however, information on only some of the uses is available, and this section cannot be considered to be comprehensive. In an effort to provide estimates of production in some European countries, the Stanford Research Institute in Zurich sent general questionnaires to some of those European companies thought to produce the compounds being evaluated. Information from the replies to these questionnaires has been compiled by country and included in the individual monographs.

Statements concerning regulations in some countries are mentioned as examples only. They may not reflect the most recent situation, since such legislation is in a constant state of change; nor should it be taken to imply that other countries do not have similar regulations. In the case of drugs, mention of the therapeutic uses of such chemicals does not necessarily represent presently accepted therapeutic indications, nor does it imply judgement as to their clinical efficacy.

The purpose of the section on analysis is to give the reader a general indication, rather than a complete review, of methods cited in the literature. No attempt is made to evaluate the methods quoted.

Biological Data Relevant to the Evaluation of Carcinogenic Risk to Man (section 3)

The monographs are not intended to consider all reported studies. Some studies were purposely omitted (a) because they were inadequate, as judged from previously described criteria[22-25] (e.g., too short a duration, too few animals, poor survival or too small a dose); (b) because they only confirmed findings which have already been fully described; or (c) because they were judged irrelevant for the purpose of the evaluation. However, in certain cases, reference is made to studies which did not meet established criteria of adequacy, particularly when this information was considered a useful supplement to other reports or when it was the only data available. Their inclusion does not, however, imply acceptance of the adequacy of their experimental design.

In general, the data recorded in this section are summarized as given by the author; however, certain shortcomings of reporting or of experimental design that were commented upon by the Working Group are given in square brackets.

Carcinogenicity and related studies in animals: Mention is made of all routes of administration by which the compound has been adequately tested and of all species in which relevant tests have been carried out. In most cases, animal strains are given; general characteristics of mouse strains have been reviewed[26]. Quantitative data are given to indicate the order of magnitude of the effective doses. In general, the doses are indicated as they appear in the original paper; sometimes conversions have been made for better comparison. When the carcinogenicity of known metabolites has been tested this also is reported.

Other relevant biological data: LD_{50} data are given when available, and other data on toxicity are included when considered relevant. The metabolic data included is restricted to studies showing the metabolic fate of the chemical in animals and man, and comparisons of animal and human data are made when possible. Other metabolic information (e.g.,

16

absorption, storage and excretion) is given when the Working Group considered that it would be useful for the reader to have a better understanding of the fate of the compound in the body.

Teratogenicity data from studies in experimental animals and in humans are included for some of the substances considered, however, they are not meant to represent a thorough review of the literature.

Mutagenicity data are also included; the reasons for including them and the principles adopted by the Working Group for their selection are outlined below.

Many, but not all, mutagens are carcinogens and *vice versa*; the exact level of correlation is still under investigation. Nevertheless, practical use may be made of the available mutagenicity test procedures that combine microbial, mammalian or other animal cell systems as genetic targets with an *in vitro* or *in vivo* metabolic activation system. The results of relatively rapid and inexpensive mutagenicity tests on non-human organisms may help to pre-screen chemicals and may also aid in the selection of the most relevant animal species in which to carry out long-term carcinogenicity tests on these chemicals.

The role of genetic alterations in chemical carcinogenesis is not yet fully understood, and therefore consideration must be given to a variety of changes. Although nuclear DNA has been defined as the main cellular target for the induction of genetic changes, other relevant targets have been recognized, e.g., mitochondrial DNA, enzymes involved in DNA synthesis, repair and recombination, and the spindle apparatus. Tests to detect the genetic activity of chemicals, including gene mutation, structural and numerical chromosomal changes and mitotic recombination, are available for non-human models; but not all such tests can be applied at present to human cells.

Ideally, an appropriate mutagenicity test system would include the full metabolic competency of the intact human.Since the development or appli-cation of such a system appears to be impossible, a battery of test systems is necessary in order to establish the mutagenic potential of chemicals. There are many genetic indicators and metabolic activation systems available for detecting mutagenic activity; they all, however, have individual advantages and limitations.

Since many chemicals require metabolism to an active form, test systems which do not take this into account may fail to reveal the full range of genetic damage. Furthermore, since some reactive metabolites with a limited lifespan may fail to reach or to react with the genetic indicator, either because they are further metabolized to inactive compounds or because they react with other cellular constituents, mutagenicity tests in intact animals may give false negative results.

It is difficult in the present state of knowledge to select specific mutagenicity tests as being the most appropriate for the pre-screening of substances for possible carcinogenic activity. However, greater reliance may be placed on data obtained from those test systems which (a) permit identification of the nature of induced genetic changes, and (b) demonstrate that the changes are transmitted to subsequent generations. Mutagenicity tests using organisms that are well-understood genetically, e.g., *Escherichia coli*, *Salmonella typhimurium*, *Saccharomyces* and *Drosophila*, meet these requirements.

Although a correlation has often been observed between the ability of a chemical to cause chromosome breakage and its ability to induce gene mutation, data on chromosomal breakage alone do not provide adequate evidence for mutagenicity, and therefore less weight should be given to pre-screening that is based on the use of peripheral leucocyte cultures.

Because of the complexity of factors that can contribute to reproductive failure, as well as the insensitivity of the method, the dominant lethal test in the mammal does not provide reliable data on mutagenicity.

A large-scale systematic screening of compounds to assess a correlation between mutagenicity and carcinogenicity has so far been carried out only with the bacterial/mammalian liver microsome system. Notwithstanding the demonstration of the mutagenicity of many known carcinogens to *Salmonella typhimurium* in the presence of liver microsomal systems, the possibility of false-negative and false-positive results must not be overlooked. False negatives might arise as a consequence of mutagen specificity or from failure to achieve optimal conditions for activation *in vitro*. Alternative test systems must be used if there appear to be substantial reasons for suspecting that a chemical which is apparently non-mutagenic in a bacterial test system may nevertheless be potentially carcinogenic. Conversely, some chemicals found to be mutagenic in this test may not in fact have mutagenic activity in other systems.

For more detailed information, see references 27-34.

Observations in man: Case reports of cancer and epidemiological studies are summarized in this section.

Comments on Data Reported and Evaluation (section 4)

This section gives the critical view of the Working Group on the data reported.

Animal data: The animal species mentioned are those in which the carcinogenicity of the substances was clearly demonstrated. The route of administration used in experimental animals that is similar to the possible human exposure (ingestion, inhalation and skin exposure) is given particular mention. Tumour sites are also indicated.

Experiments involving a possible action of the vehicle or a physical effect of the agent, such as in studies by subcutaneous injection or bladder implantation, are included; however, the results of such tests require careful consideration, particularly if they are the only ones raising a suspicion of carcinogenicity. If the substance has produced tumours after pre-natal exposure or in single-dose experiments, this also is indicated. This sub-section should be read in the light of comments made in the section, 'Animal Data in Relation to the Evaluation of Risk to Man' of this introduction.

Human data: In some cases, a brief statement is made on possible human exposure. The significance of epidemiological studies and case reports is discussed, and the data are interpreted in terms of possible human risk.

References

1. IARC (1972) <u>IARC Monographs on the Evaluation of Carcinogenic Risk of Chemicals to Man</u>, <u>1</u>, Lyon

2. IARC (1973) <u>IARC Monographs on the Evaluation of Carcinogenic Risk of Chemicals to Man</u>, <u>2</u>, <u>Some Inorganic and Organometallic Compounds</u>, Lyon

3. IARC (1973) <u>IARC Monographs on the Evaluation of Carcinogenic Risk of Chemicals to Man</u>, <u>3</u>, <u>Certain Polycyclic Aromatic Hydrocarbons and Heterocyclic Compounds</u>, Lyon

4. IARC (1974) <u>IARC Monographs on the Evaluation of Carcinogenic Risk of Chemicals to Man</u>, <u>4</u>, <u>Some Aromatic Amines, Hydrazine and Related Substances, N-Nitroso Compounds and Miscellaneous Alkylating Agents</u>, Lyon

5. IARC (1974) <u>IARC Monographs on the Evaluation of Carcinogenic Risk of Chemicals to Man</u>, <u>5</u>, <u>Some Organochlorine Pesticides</u>, Lyon

6. IARC (1974) <u>IARC Monographs on the Evaluation of Carcinogenic Risk of Chemicals to Man</u>, <u>6</u>, <u>Sex Hormones</u>, Lyon

7. IARC (1974) <u>IARC Monographs on the Evaluation of Carcinogenic Risk of Chemicals to Man</u>, <u>7</u>, <u>Some Anti-thyroid and Related Substances, Nitrofurans and Industrial Chemicals</u>, Lyon

8. IARC (1975) <u>IARC Monographs on the Evaluation of Carcinogenic Risk of Chemicals to Man</u>, <u>8</u>, <u>Some Aromatic Azo Compounds</u>, Lyon

9. IARC (1975) <u>IARC Monographs on the Evaluation of Carcinogenic Risk of Chemicals to Man</u>, <u>9</u>, <u>Some Aziridines, N-, S- and O-Mustards and Selenium</u>, Lyon

10. IARC (1976) <u>IARC Monographs on the Evaluation of Carcinogenic Risk of Chemicals to Man</u>, <u>10</u>, <u>Some Naturally Occurring Substances</u>, Lyon

11. IARC (1976) <u>IARC Monographs on the Evaluation of Carcinogenic Risk of Chemicals to Man</u>, <u>11</u>, <u>Cadmium, Nickel, Some Epoxides, Miscellaneous Industrial Chemicals and General Considerations on Volatile Anaesthetics</u>, Lyon

12. IARC (1976) <u>IARC Monographs on the Evaluation of Carcinogenic Risk of Chemicals to Man</u>, <u>12</u>, <u>Some Carbamates, Thiocarbamates and Carbazides</u>, Lyon

13. Hartwell, J.L. (1951) <u>Survey of Compounds which have been Tested for Carcinogenic Activity</u>, Washington DC, US Government Printing Office (Public Health Service Publication No. 149)

14. Shubik, P. & Hartwell, J.L. (1957) Survey of Compounds which have been Tested for Carcinogenic Activity, Washington DC, US Government Printing Office (Public Health Service Publication No. 149: Supplement 1)

15. Shubik, P. & Hartwell, J.L. (1969) Survey of Compounds which have been Tested for Carcinogenic Activity, Washington DC, US Government Printing Office (Public Health Service Publication No. 149: Supplement 2)

16. Carcinogenesis Program National Cancer Institute (1971) Survey of Compounds which have been Tested for Carcinogenic Activity, Washington DC, US Government Printing Office (Public Health Service Publication No. 149: 1968-1969)

17. Carcinogenesis Program National Cancer Institute (1973) Survey of Compounds which have been Tested for Carcinogenic Activity, Washington DC, US Government Printing Office (Public Health Service Publication No. 149: 1961-1967)

18. Carcinogenesis Program National Cancer Institute (1974) Survey of Compounds which have been Tested for Carcinogenic Activity, Washington DC, US Government Printing Office (Public Health Service Publication No. 149: 1970-1971)

19. WHO (1961) Fifth Report of the Joint FAO/WHO Expert Committee on Food Additives. Evaluation of carcinogenic hazard of food additives. Wld Hlth Org. techn. Rep. Ser., No. 220, pp. 5, 18, 19

20. WHO (1969) Report of a WHO Scientific Group. Principles for the testing and evaluation of drugs for carcinogenicity. Wld Hlth Org. techn. Rep. Ser., No. 426, pp. 19, 21, 22

21. WHO (1964) Report of a WHO Expert Committee. Prevention of cancer. Wld Hlth Org. techn. Rep. Ser., No. 276, pp. 29, 30

22. WHO (1958) Second Report of the Joint FAO/WHO Expert Committee on Food Additives. Procedures for the testing of intentional food additives to establish their safety for use. Wld Hlth Org. techn. Rep. Ser., No. 144

23. WHO (1961) Fifth Report of the Joint FAO/WHO Expert Committee on Food Additives. Evaluation of carcinogenic hazard of food additives. Wld Hlth Org. techn. Rep. Ser., No. 220

24. WHO (1967) Scientific Group. Procedures for investigating intentional and unintentional food additives. Wld Hlth Org. techn. Rep. Ser., No. 348

25. Berenblum, I., ed. (1969) Carcinogenicity testing. UICC techn. Rep. Ser., 2

26. Committee on Standardized Genetic Nomenclature for Mice (1972) Standardized nomenclature for inbred strains of mice. Fifth listing. Cancer Res., 32, 1609-1646

27. Bartsch, H. & Grover, P.L. (1976) Chemical carcinogenesis and mutagenesis. In: Symington, T. & Carter, R.L., eds, Scientific Foundations of Oncology, Vol. IX, Chemical Carcinogenesis, London, Heinemann Medical Books Ltd, pp. 334-342

28. Holländer, A., ed. (1971) Chemical Mutagens: Principles and Methods for Their Detection, Vols 1-3, New York, Plenum Press

29. Montesano, R. & Tomatis, L., eds (1974) Chemical Carcinogenesis Essays, Lyon (IARC Scientific Publications No. 10)

30. Ramel, C., ed. (1973) Evaluation of genetic risks of environmental chemicals: report of a symposium held at Skokloster, Sweden, 1972. Ambio Special Report, No. 3

31. Stoltz, D.R., Poirier, L.A., Irving, C.C., Stich, H.F., Weisburger, J.H. & Grice, H.C. (1974) Evaluation of short-term tests for carcinogenicity. Toxicol. appl. Pharmacol., 29, 157-180

32. WHO (1974) Report of WHO Scientific Group. Assessment of the carcinogenicity and mutagenicity of chemicals. Wld Hlth Org. techn. Rep. Ser., No. 546

33. Montesano, R., Bartsch, H. & Tomatis, L., eds (1976) Screening Tests in Chemical Carcinogenesis, Lyon (IARC Scientific Publications No. 12)

34. Committee 17 (1975) Environmental mutagenic hazards. Science, 187, 503-514

GENERAL REMARKS ON SUBSTANCES CONSIDERED

This volume includes monographs on a number of miscellaneous pharmaceutical substances for which epidemiological reports and/or animal studies suggest a possible carcinogenic activity. Although the term 'drug' is often used to describe compounds which are used illicitly, for the purposes of this volume of monographs it has been used synonymously with the term 'pharmaceutical substance'. Since only a limited number of compounds can be evaluated at any one meeting, the list of drugs reviewed here is not meant to be exhaustive. Certain other drugs have already been considered in previous volumes of monographs in this series (Vols 2, 4, 6, 7, 9 & 10).

A number of drugs were considered but eventually not included because the available data were inadequate. These drugs are: acetylsalicylic acid, amobarbital, chlorpromazine, diphenylthiohydantoin, lysergide (LSD), nitroxoline, pentobarbital sodium, prednisone, pyrazinamide, rifampicin and spironolactone. On-going carcinogenicity studies in experimental animals are in progress for many of these substances (IARC, 1976). A particular case is that of acetylsalicylic acid (aspirin), for which the available human and experimental data were insufficient to make an evaluation: the results of only two inadequate carcinogenicity tests on this very common drug were available. The Working Group was aware, however, of several on-going carcinogenicity studies on this compound. Although evidence of teratogenicity is not necessarily related to an evaluation of carcinogenicity, it is also worth noting that the experimental evidence of a teratogenic action of aspirin has not been followed up by adequate studies to confirm or exclude a similar effect in humans.

Azathioprine was also considered by this Working Group. Although experimental evidence for its carcinogenicity existed, it was felt by some members of the Working Group that it would be more appropriate to consider this compound in the context of other immunosuppressive drugs.

Some of the compounds considered are amines which, in principle, could be converted to carcinogenic N-nitroso compounds by reaction with nitrite under mildly acid conditions. It is well known that nitrate and, to a lesser extent, nitrite occur in many foods and that nitrate can be reduced to nitrite in the gastrointestinal tract. Thus, N-nitrosodialkylamines could be formed in the stomach from a number of drugs with tertiary amino groups. Drugs which contain secondary amino groups could also form the corresponding N-nitroso drugs.

Regulatory requirements that include assay, identification and limit tests for impurities in pharmaceutical grade drugs or pharmaceutical products are given in various national and international pharmacopoeias, such as the British Pharmacopoeia, The US Pharmacopeia, WHO International Pharmacopoeia and European Pharmacopoeia. Such information is given for a number of drugs considered in this volume. No attempt was made to give such requirements in detail in the section on analysis; however, these monographs describe simple and effective methods for testing the purity of both pure and formulated drugs.

When evaluating drug-cancer relationships, the following points, in addition to the possibility that the drug itself may cause the cancer, should also be considered:

(1) The pathological condition may predispose to cancer (see Table I).

(2) The cancer may predispose to the pathological condition (see Table I - Epilepsy).

(3) The pathological condition or the treatment may increase the chance of diagnosis of cancer but not cause an increase in its incidence.

(4) Some third factor (e.g., a genetic factor) may cause both the pathological condition and cancer, which are not otherwise related.

(5) The pathological condition and the cancer are, in reality, phases of the same process.

(6) Patients may be exposed to more than one drug either sequentially or in combination.

(7) Patients administered the drug may, as a consequence, survive longer.

TABLE I

Examples of associations between some pathological conditions
(in which drugs included in the present monograph are used) and cancer

Original pathological condition	Drug used	Independent associations of the original pathological condition with cancer which may confound the assessment of the relationship between drug use and cancer
Epilepsy	Phenytoin Phenobarbital	Brain tumours could cause epileptic seizures and could therefore coexist with the disease at a higher frequency than the expected rate (Clemmesen et al., 1974).
Fanconi's anaemia	Oxymetholone	One case of hepatoma has been reported in a patient with Fanconi's anaemia who was never treated with androgenic steroids (Cattan et al., 1974). Patients with Fanconi's anaemia have a high risk of developing acute leukaemia (Dosik et al., 1970).
Malaria	Chloroquine Pyrimethamine	There is an apparent connection between malaria infection and Burkitt's lymphoma (Burkitt, 1969; Dalldorf et al., 1964; IARC, 1975; O'Connor, 1970).
Schistosomiasis	Niridazole Hycanthone	There is an association between infection by *Schistosoma haematobium* and urinary bladder cancer (Edington, 1956; Hashem, 1961; Mustacchi & Shimkin, 1958). One report has discussed the association between infection by *S. mansoni* and lymphoma in man (Andrade & Abreu, 1971).
Trichomoniasis	Metronidazole	The incidence of trichomonal infection in 3682 non-gynaecological in-patients with negative (Class I and II) smears was 10%. Trichomonal infection was present in 35% of patients with dysplasia of the cervix, carcinoma *in situ* or adenocarcinoma of the uterus (Wachtel et al., 1972). Berggren (1969) and Bertini & Hornstein (1970) found an increased incidence of trichomonal infection in patients with malignant and premalignant diseases of the cervix. An association between herpes simplex virus type 2 and cervical carcinoma *in situ* has also been established (Nahmias et al., 1974).

25

References

Andrade, Z.A. & Abreu, W.N. (1971) Follicular lymphoma of the spleen in patients with hepatosplenic schistosomiasis mansoni. Amer. J. trop. Med. Hyg., 20, 237-243

Berggren, O. (1969) Association of carcinoma of the uterine cervix and *Trichomonas vaginalis* infestations. Amer. J. Obstet. Gynec., 105, 166-168

Bertini, B. & Hornstein, M. (1970) The epidemiology of trichomoniasis and the role of this infection in the development of carcinoma of the cervix. Acta cytol., 14, 325-332

Burkitt, D.P. (1969) Etiology of Burkitt's lymphoma - an alternative hypothesis to a vectored virus. J. nat. Cancer Inst., 42, 19-28

Cattan, D., Kalifat, F., Wautier, J.-L., Meignan, S., Vesin, P. & Piet, R. (1974) Maladie de Fanconi et cancer du foie. Arch. franç. Mal. App. Dig., 63, 41-48

Clemmesen, J., Fuglsang-Frederiksen, V. & Plum, C.M. (1974) Are anticonvulsants oncogenic? Lancet, i, 705-707

Dalldorf, G., Linsell, C.A., Barnhart, F.E. & Martyn, R. (1964) An epidemiologic approach to the lymphomas of African children and Burkitt's sarcoma of the jaws. Perspect. Biol. Med., 7, 435-449

Dosik, H., Hsu, L.Y., Todaro, G.J., Lee, S.L., Hirschhorn, K., Selirio, E.S. & Alter, A.A. (1970) Leukemia in Fanconi's anemia: cytogenetic and tumor virus susceptibility studies. Blood, 36, 341-352

Edington, G.M. (1956) Malignant disease in the Gold Coast. Brit. J. Cancer, 10, 595-608

Hashem, M. (1961) The aetiology and pathogenesis of the bilharzial bladder cancer. J. Egypt. med. Ass., 44, 857-966

IARC (1975) Annual Report, 1975, Lyon, International Agency for Research on Cancer, pp. 15-16

IARC (1976) IARC Information Bulletin on the Survey of Chemicals Being Tested for Carcinogenicity, No. 6, Lyon

Mustacchi, P. & Shimkin, M.B. (1958) Cancer of the bladder and infestation with *Schistosoma hematobium*. J. nat. Cancer Inst., 20, 825-842

Nahmias, A.J., Naib, Z.M. & Josey, W.E. (1974) Epidemiological studies relating genital herpetic infection to cervical carcinoma. Cancer Res., 34, 1111-1117

O'Connor, G.T. (1970) Persistent immunologic stimulation as a factor in oncogenesis, with special reference to Burkitt's tumor. Amer. J. Med. 48, 279-285

Wachtel, E., Wycherley, J. & Lee, C.N. (1972) Screening for cancer of the female genital tract in general medical and surgical wards. Practitioner, 208, 505-508

THE MONOGRAPHS

ACRIFLAVINIUM CHLORIDE

1. Chemical and Physical Data

1.1 Synonyms and trade names

Chem. Abstr. Reg. Serial No.: 8048-52-0

Chem. Abstr. Name: 3,6-Diamino-10-methylacridinium chloride mixture with 3,6-acridinediamine

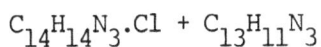

Acriflavine mixture with proflavine; acriflavinii chloridum; 3,6-diaminoacridine mixture with 3,6-diamino-10-methylacridinium chloride; 2,8-diamino-10-methylacridinium chloride mixture with 2,8-diaminoacridine; flavacridinum hydrochloricum; neutral acriflavine; neutroflavine; trypaflavine; trypaflavine neutral; trypaflavinum; xanthacridinum

Acriflavon; Angiflan; Assiflavine; Avlon; Bialflavina; Bioacridin; Bovoflavin; Burnol; Buroflavin; Choliflavin; Chromoflavine; Diacrid; Euflavin; Euflavine; Flaviform; Flavine; Flavinetten; Flavipin; Flavisept; Glyco-Flavine; Gonacin; Gonacrine; Isravin; Mediflavin; Neutroflavin; Panflavin; Pantonsiletten; Tolivalin; Trachosept; Tripla-Etilo; Trypaflavin; Vetaflavin; Zoriflavin

1.2 Chemical formulae and molecular weight

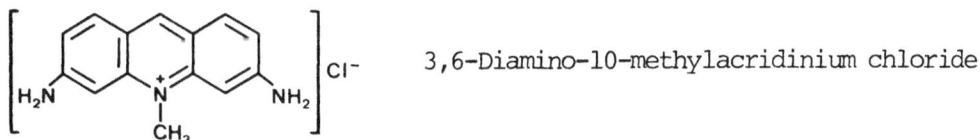

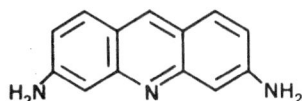

3,6-Diamino-10-methylacridinium chloride

3,6-Acridinediamine

$$C_{14}H_{14}N_3 \cdot Cl + C_{13}H_{11}N_3 \qquad \text{Mol. wt: } 469.0$$

1.3 Chemical and physical properties of the pure substance

From Gupta *et al.* (1967), unless otherwise specified

(a) Description: Red microcrystals

(b) Melting-point: 295-298°C

(c) Spectroscopy data: λ_{max} 261 nm (E_1^1 = 1337) and 465 nm (E_1^1 = 1531) in ethanol

(d) Solubility: Soluble in water, 33 g/100 ml; slightly soluble in ethanol; nearly insoluble in chloroform, ether and fixed oils (Stecher, 1968)

1.4 Technical products and impurities

Acriflavinium chloride is a mixture of acriflavine and proflavine and can be obtained in the US in a mixture stated to contain as much as 30% proflavine (Gupta *et al.*, 1967).

2. Production, Use, Occurrence and Analysis

For important background information on this section, see preamble, p. 15.

2.1 Production and use

(a) Production

Acriflavinium chloride was synthesized in 1910 by Ehrlich and Benda. It can be prepared by heating *meta*-phenylenediamine with oxalic acid, glycerol and a condensing agent, followed by methylation with dimethyl sulphate or methyl *para*-toluenesulphonate (The Society of Dyers and Colourists, 1971).

Acriflavinium chloride has been produced commercially in the US for over 50 years (US Tariff Commission, 1927); only one US company reported production (see preamble, p. 15) in 1972 (US Tariff Commission, 1974a). US imports of acriflavinium chloride through the principal customs districts were reported to be 380 kg in 1972 (US Tariff Commission, 1973), 255 kg in 1973 (US Tariff Commission, 1974b) and 240 kg in 1974 (US International Trade Commission, 1976).

No evidence has been found that acriflavinium chloride is produced commercially in Japan; 250 kg were imported from the Federal Republic of Germany in 1975. It is produced by at least one company in Europe; however, annual production estimates were not available.

(b) Use

Acriflavinium chloride has been used as a topical antiseptic, due to its bacteriostatic action (Klarmann, 1963), and as a urinary antiseptic (Stecher, 1968); for topical use a 0.01-0.1% solution is usually applied (Stecher, 1968).

It has been used in Japan in the treatment of gonorrhoea, and in the USSR in the treatment of meningitis, endocarditis and St Anthony's Fire (herpes zoster) (Mashkovski, 1972).

Acriflavinium chloride was formerly used in veterinary medicine as an udder infusion in bovine mastitis, to treat trichomonal infections in bulls and in piroplasmosis. It has reportedly been used locally in wounds (Stecher, 1968).

It has also been used as a basic dye but is no longer in commercial use for that purpose (The Society of Dyers and Colourists, 1971).

2.2 Occurrence

Acriflavinium chloride is not known to occur in nature.

2.3 Analysis

Determinations of acriflavinium chloride involve chromatographic separation techniques, including column and paper chromatography and paper electrophoresis, prior to spectrophotometric analysis (Gupta et al., 1967). Thin-layer chromatographic methods have been developed (Thielemann, 1973) and include a method using partition and ion-exchange thin-layer chromatography on cellulose (Gill, 1967).

3. Biological Data Relevant to the Evaluation
of Carcinogenic Risk to Man

3.1 Carcinogenicity and related studies in animals

Subcutaneous administration

Rat: A group of 24 young, adult, random-bred white rats of both sexes received s.c. injections of 1 mg acriflavinium chloride/animal in 0.4 ml olive oil at 15-day intervals (total dose, 40 mg/animal). At 12 months, 14 animals were still alive, and the experiment was terminated 20 months after the first injection, at which time 3 rats remained alive. One animal developed a sarcoma at the site of injection 14 months after the beginning of the treatment. No tumours occurred in 20 controls receiving olive oil alone (Ezeyza, 1952).

3.2 Other relevant biological data

(a) Experimental systems

The s.c. lethal dose of acriflavinium chloride in mice is 250 mg/kg bw (Stecher, 1968). After administration of i.p. doses of 10 or 30 mg/kg bw or of 50 mg/kg bw orally in male mice, the compound could be detected in germ cells (Baldermann et al., 1967).

Acriflavinium chloride interacts with DNA in HeLa cells and in SV40 virus-transformed mouse cells (Smith et al., 1971). Studies with isolated DNA on the mechanism of acriflavinium chloride-DNA interaction have included flow dichroism studies with calf thymus DNA (Nagata et al., 1966) and fluorescence-quenching studies with synthetic polynucleotides (Schreiber & Daune, 1974).

Acriflavinium chloride induces point mutations in Escherichia coli (Demerec et al., 1947). It is a weak inducer of frame-shift mutations in Salmonella typhimurium his-C_{3076}, without metabolic activation (Tosk, 1974), and a stronger frame-shift mutagen in TA98 and TA1537 in the presence of rat liver homogenates (Brown & Brown, 1976). It induces respiratory-deficient petite mutants in Saccharomyces cerevisiae (Bień, 1972; Bień & Konrad, 1972). At high oral doses (50 mg/kg bw) in male mice, it was weakly positive in the dominant lethal test (Baldermann et al., 1967); at lower doses given by i.p. injection it was negative (Baldermann *et al.*, 1967; Epstein *et al.*, 1972).

(b) Man

Acriflavinium chloride induces altered sedimentation velocity of DNA from cultured human fibroblasts (Kleijer *et al.*, 1973) and binds to DNA in cultured buccal cells (Roth, 1971; Roth & Manjon, 1969).

Chromosome abnormalities in HeLa cells and cultured peripheral human leucocytes have been reported at a concentration of 10^{-6} M/l in the absence of light; at 10^{-9}-10^{-7} M/l, chromosome abnormalities were observed in both HeLa cells and in peripheral leucocytes on exposure for 1 hour to light (Buchinger, 1969).

3.3 Case reports and epidemiological studies

No data were available to the Working Group.

4. Comments on Data Reported and Evaluation

4.1 Animal data

No evaluation concerning the carcinogenicity of acriflavinium chloride can be made from the only limited study in rats given the compound by subcutaneous injection. Further testing of this compound would appear to be desirable, also in view of the results obtained in mutagenicity studies.

4.2 Human data

No case reports or epidemiological studies were available to the Working Group.

5. References

Baldermann, K.H., Röhrborn, G. & Schroeder, T.M. (1967) Mutagenitäts-untersuchungen mit Trypaflavin und Hexamethylentetramin am Säuger *in vivo* und *in vitro*. Humangenetik, 4, 112-126

Bień, M. (1972) Sensitivity of *Saccharomyces cerevisiae* in various phases of the life cycle to induction by acriflavine. II. Induction of mutants by acriflavine in diploid cultures. Acta microbiol. pol., Ser. A, 4, 91-98

Bień, M. & Konrad, B. (1972) Sensitivity of *Saccharomyces cerevisiae* in various phases of the life cycle to induction by acriflavine. III. Induction of mutants during sporulation. Acta microbiol. pol., Ser. A, 4, 99-106

Brown, J.P. & Brown, R.J. (1976) Mutagenesis by 9,10-anthraquinone derivatives and related compounds in *Salmonella typhimurium*. Mutation Res., 40, 203-224

Buchinger, G. (1969) Die Wirkung von Trypaflavin allein und in Kombination mit sichtbaren Licht auf die Chromosomen von HeLa-Zellen und mensch-liche Leukocyten. Humangenetik, 7, 323-336

Demerec, M., Witkin, E.M., Newcombe, H.B. & Beale, G.H. (1947) The gene. Carnegie Institution Wash. Yearbook, 46, 127-135

Epstein, S.S., Arnold, E., Andrea, J., Bass, W. & Bishop, Y. (1972) Detection of chemical mutagens by the dominant lethal assay in the mouse. Toxicol. appl. Pharmacol., 23, 288-325

Ezeyza, S. (1952) Neosalvarsán, sulfato de atropina y tripaflavina en ratas inyectadas subcutáneamente: carencia de poder cancerígeno de los dos primeros y producción de un sarcoma en el lugar de la inyección de tripaflavina. Semana méd., 100, 778-780

Gill, J.E. (1967) Partition and ion-exchange thin-layer chromatography of water-soluble fluorescent compounds. J. Chromat., 26, 315-319

Gupta, V.S., Kraft, S.C. & Samuelson, J.S. (1967) Purification and properties of acriflavine, proflavine and related compounds. J. Chromat., 26, 158-163

Klarmann, E.G. (1963) Antiseptics and disinfectants. In: Kirk, R.E. & Othmer, D.F., eds, Encyclopedia of Chemical Technology, 2nd ed., Vol. 2, New York, John Wiley and Sons, p. 639

Kleijer, W.J., Hoeksema, J.L., Sluyter, M.L. & Bootsma, D. (1973) Effects of inhibitors on repair of DNA in normal human and xeroderma pigmento-sum cells after exposure to X-rays and ultraviolet radiation. Mutation Res., 17, 385-394

Mashkovski, M.D. (1972) Drug Compounds, Vol. 2, Moscow, Medizina, p. 465

Nagata, C., Kodama, M., Tagashira, Y. & Imamura, A. (1966) Interaction of polynuclear aromatic hydrocarbons, 4-nitroquinoline 1-oxides, and various dyes with DNA. Biopolymers, 4, 409-427

Roth, D. (1971) An acridine label for thymine photodimers in intact cells. EMS Newslett., 4, 38-39

Roth, D. & Manjon, M.L. (1969) Studies of a specific association between acriflavine and DNA in intact cells. Biopolymers, 7, 695-705

Schreiber, J.P. & Daune, M.P. (1974) Fluorescence of complexes of acridine dye with synthetic polydeoxyribonucleotides: a physical model of frameshift mutation. J. mol. Biol., 83, 487-501

Smith, C.A., Jordan, J.M. & Vinograd, J. (1971) In vivo effects of intercalating drugs on the superhelix density of mitochondrial DNA isolated from human and mouse cells in culture. J. mol. Biol., 59, 255-272

The Society of Dyers and Colourists (1971) Colour Index, 3rd ed., Vol. 4, Bradford, Yorks, p. 4431

Stecher, P.G., ed. (1968) The Merck Index, 8th ed., Rahway, NJ, Merck & Co., p. 16

Thielemann, H. (1973) Dünnschichtchromatographische Trennung und Identifizierung von Acriflavin (3,6-Diamino-10-methylacridinium-hydroxyd) und Äthacridin (2-Äthoxy-6,9-diaminoacridin-lactat). Sci. Pharm., 41, 338-339

Tosk, J. (1974) Chlorpromazine protection against acridine-induced reversion of a histidine-requiring mutant of Salmonella typhimurium. Mutation Res., 24, 1-3

US International Trade Commission (1976) Imports of Benzenoid Chemicals and Products, 1974, USITC Publication 762, Washington DC, US Government Printing Office, p. 79

US Tariff Commission (1927) Census of Dyes and Other Synthetic Organic Chemicals, 1926, Tariff Information Series No. 35, Washington DC, US Government Printing Office, p. 70

US Tariff Commission (1973) Imports of Benzenoid Chemicals and Products, 1972, TC Publication 601, Washington DC, US Government Printing Office, p. 82

US Tariff Commission (1974a) Synthetic Organic Chemicals, US Production and Sales, 1972, TC Publication 681, Washington DC, US Government Printing Office, p. 110

US Tariff Commission (1974b) Imports of Benzenoid Chemicals and Products, 1973, TC Publication 688, Washington DC, US Government Printing Office, p. 78

AUROTHIOGLUCOSE

1. Chemical and Physical Data

1.1 Synonyms and trade names

Chem. Abstr. Reg. Serial No.: 12192-57-3

Chem. Abstr. Name: (1-Thio-D-glucopyranosato)gold

1-Aurothio-D-glucopyranose; (D-glucopyranosylthio)gold; (1-D-glucosylthio)gold; gold thioglucose; (1-thio-D-glucopyrano-sato)gold; 1-thio-D-glucopyranose, gold complex; 1-thio-gluco-pyranose, monogold(1+)salt; 1-thio-D-glucopyranose, monogold(1+)salt

Aureotan; Auromyose; Aurumine; Authron; Brenol; Glysanol B; Oronol; Romosol; Solganal; Solganal B; Solganol B

1.2 Chemical formula and molecular weight

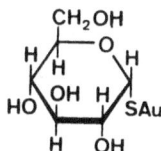

$C_6H_{11}AuO_5S$ Mol. wt: 392.2

1.3 Chemical and physical properties of the pure substance

From Stecher (1968)

(a) Description: Yellow crystals

(b) Solubility: Soluble in water with decomposition; slightly soluble in propylene glycol; insoluble in ethanol, in most other organic solvents and in vegetable oils

1.4 Technical products and impurities

Aurothioglucose is available in the US as a USP grade containing 95-105.0% active ingredient on a dried basis; it is stabilized with small amounts of no more than 5% sodium acetate (Harvey, 1975). Ampoules containing 50 or 100 mg aurothioglucose/ml as a sterile suspension in a suitable vegetable oil are also available and contain 90-110% of the stated amount of aurothioglucose. Suitable thickening agents may also be present in the suspension (US Pharmacopeial Convention, Inc., 1975).

2. Production, Use, Occurrence and Analysis

For important background information on this section, see preamble, p. 15.

2.1 Production and use

(a) Production

Aurothioglucose can be prepared by refluxing gold tribromide with an aqueous solution of thioglucose in the presence of sulphur dioxide (Harvey, 1975).

Commercial production of aurothioglucose in the US was first reported in 1940 (US Tariff Commission, 1941); only one US company reported production (see preamble, p.) in 1974 (US International Trade Commission, 1976). No evidence was found that it has ever been produced commercially or imported in Japan. No data were available concerning its production in Europe. .

(b) Use

The chief therapeutic application of aurothioglucose is in rheumatoid arthritis (Harvey, 1970). However, the vast majority of such patients are treated with acetylsalicylic acid and newer anti-inflammatory drugs; aurothioglucose is reserved for the treatment of more severe cases resistant to other modes of treatment. For active rheumatoid arthritis, a suggested dose schedule involves i.m. administration of 10, then 25, then 50 mg weekly until a total dose of 800-1,000 mg has been given, followed by 50 mg every second or third week for 4 doses, then monthly thereafter (Harvey, 1975).

Aurothioglucose is used to a lesser extent in the treatment of non-disseminated lupus erythematosus (Harvey, 1970).

It has been used experimentally in veterinary practice to produce obesity (Stecher, 1968).

2.2 Occurrence

Aurothioglucose is not known to occur in nature.

2.3 Analysis

Aurothioglucose in bulk and injection form can be determined gravimetrically (US Pharmacopeial Convention, Inc., 1975). It can be analysed by anodic stripping voltammetry (Schmid & Bolger, 1973), and a colorimetric determination has been developed (Janik & Rzeszutko, 1969).

3. Biological Data Relevant to the Evaluation of Carcinogenic Risk to Man

3.1 Carcinogenicity and related studies in animals

Intraperitoneal administration

Mouse: A group of 88 8-12-week old virgin female C3H mice receiving an unrestricted diet **were** given single i.p. injections of 10 mg/animal aurothioglucose; 78/88 mice became obese following this treatment. At 295 days, 50% of these mice developed mammary tumours, compared with 354 days in 50% of untreated controls; after 295 days only 19% of 66 controls had mammary tumours. The 10 treated mice that did not become obese developed mammary tumours within a time similar to that in controls (Waxler et al., 1953).

Mammary tumours developed in 38/38 virgin female RIIIxCBA mice that became obese after receiving a single i.p. injection of 400 mg/kg bw at 70-80 days of age, compared with 29/34 untreated virgin females (controls) and 10/10 untreated breeders. Fifty percent of the animals in the three groups developed mammary tumours at 240, 350 and 250 days, respectively. The average numbers of tumours per animal were 3.2 in aurothioglucose-treated virgin females, 1.9 in controls and 2.2 in untreated breeders (Liebelt, 1959).

In groups of male and female AKR mice, thymectomized at the age of 4 weeks and given single i.p. injections of 750 mg/kg bw aurothioglucose at 10 weeks of age, 1/9 (11%) males and 5/12 (41%) females developed benign

41

osteomas of the skull, compared with 0/15 male and 1/23 (4%) female AKR thymectomized controls. Of 31 thymectomized males given a s.c. implant (amount unstated) of a cholesterol pellet containing 10% oestradiol at 14 weeks of age, 14 (45%) developed osteomas. Of 11 similarly treated males receiving in addition single i.p. injections of 750 mg/kg bw aurothioglucose, 8 (72%) developed osteomas. No osteomas occurred in similarly treated C57BL mice (Rudali, 1968).

Groups of intact (34 male and 23 female) or castrated (25 male and 22 female) CBA mice were given 400 mg/kg bw aurothioglucose in saline by i.p. injection at the age of 13-14 weeks and observed until they were 56 weeks of age; similar groups of intact (36 male and 40 female) and castrated (16 male and 15 female) controls were used. In treated animals a significant increase in the incidence of hepatomas was observed in intact males (21/34 *versus* 7/36) but not in intact females. Treated castrated males had no significant increase in the incidence of hepatomas. The 2 treated intact females that developed hepatomas also had androgen-secreting adrenal cortical tumours. The 3 untreated castrated and the 8 treated castrated males that developed hepatomas also had adrenal cortical adenomas, which were associated with androgenic activity in 8 cases (Gray *et al.*, 1960).

3.2 Other relevant biological data

(a) Experimental systems

The i.p. LD$_{50}$ of aurothioglucose in stock mice is 2000-2500 mg/kg bw (Brecher & Waxler, 1949). Doses of 350 mg/kg bw to CBA mice cause bilateral hypothalamic lesions associated with obesity; in C57BL mice doses of 1200 mg/kg bw are required to cause similar changes in weight gain (Liebelt & Perry, 1957). In Swiss mice, doses of 650 mg/kg bw caused hypothalamic lesions, but only 30% of the animals became obese (Brecher *et al.*, 1965).

Wistar rats of both sexes and of various ages showed no signs of obesity within 60-70 days after single i.p. or i.m. injections of 0.5-1.6 g/kg bw (Talbert & Hamilton, 1954). In Long-Evans rats given 400 mg/kg bw i.p., no obesity occurred, but severe hypothalamic lesions were seen (Wagner & de Groot, 1963).

In rats given i.m. injections of aurothioglucose daily for 14 days
(total dose, 14 mg gold/animal), retention of absorbed gold was greatest
in the kidney and then in the liver and spleen; 15% of the dose was
retained in the body after 85 days (Block *et al.*, 1944).

(b) Man

Water-soluble gold salts are absorbed rapidly after their i.m. injection
in humans. Approximately 85% of the injected gold is retained over 7 days.
It is excreted mainly by the kidney, but a small amount appears in the
faeces (Harvey, 1970).

3.3 Case reports and epidemiological studies

No data were available to the Working Group.

4. Comments on Data Reported and Evaluation[1]

4.1 Animal data

Aurothioglucose is carcinogenic in mice after its administration
by single intraperitoneal injection: it produced an increased incidence
of hepatomas in male mice.

4.2 Human data

No case reports or epidemiological studies were available to the
Working Group.

---

[1]See also the section 'Animal Data in Relation to the Evaluation of
Risk to Man' in the introduction to this volume, p. 13.

5. References

Block, W.D., Buchanan, O.H. & Freyberg, R.H. (1944) Metabolism, toxicity, and manner of action of gold compounds used in the treatment of arthritis. V. A comparative study of the rate of absorption, the retention, and the rate of excretion of gold administered in different compounds. J. Pharmacol. exp. Ther., 82, 391-398

Brecher, G. & Waxler, S.H. (1949) Obesity in albino mice due to single injections of goldthioglucose. Proc. Soc. exp. Biol. (N.Y.), 70, 498-501

Brecher, G., Laqueur, G.L., Cronkite, E.P., Edelman, P.M. & Schwartz, I.L. (1965) The brain lesion of goldthioglucose obesity. J. exp. Med., 121, 395-401

Gray, G.F., Liebelt, R.A. & Liebelt, A.G. (1960) The development of liver tumors in goldthioglucose-treated CBA mice. Cancer Res., 20, 1101-1104

Harvey, S.C. (1970) Heavy metals. In: Goodman, L.S. & Gilman, A., eds, The Pharmacological Basis of Therapeutics, 4th ed., New York, Macmillan, pp. 969-974

Harvey, S.C. (1975) Hormones. In: Osol, A. *et al.*, eds, Remington's Pharmaceutical Sciences, 15th ed., Easton, Pa, Mack, p. 899

Janik, B. & Rzeszutko, W. (1969) Colorimetric determination of gold in Solganal B. Acta pol. pharm., 26, 339-342

Liebelt, R.A. (1959) Effects of goldthioglucose-induced hypothalamic lesions on mammary tumorigenesis in RIIIxCBA mice. Proc. Amer. Ass. Cancer Res., 3, 37-38

Liebelt, R.A. & Perry, J.H. (1957) Hypothalamic lesions associated with goldthioglucose-induced obesity. Proc. Soc. exp. Biol. (N.Y.), 95, 774-777

Rudali, G. (1968) Apparition d'ostéomes intracraniens chez des souris injectées avec du thioglucose d'or. Rev. franç. Etud. clin. biol., 13, 40-48

Schmid, G.M. & Bolger, G.W. (1973) Determination of gold in drugs and serum by use of anodic stripping voltammetry. Clin. Chem., 19, 1002-1005

Stecher, P.G., ed. (1968) The Merck Index, 8th ed., Rahway, NJ, Merck & Co., p. 112

Talbert, G.B. & Hamilton, J.B. (1954) Failure to produce obesity in the rat following gold thioglucose injection. Proc. Soc. exp. Biol. (N.Y.), 86, 376-378

US International Trade Commission (1976) Synthetic Organic Chemicals, US Production and Sales, 1974, USITC Publication 776, Washington DC, US Government Printing Office, p. 105

US Pharmacopeial Convention, Inc. (1975) The US Pharmacopeia, 19th rev., Rockville, Md, pp. 41-42

US Tariff Commission (1941) Synthetic Organic Chemicals, US Production and Sales, 1940, Report No. 148, Second Series, Washington DC, US Government Printing Office, p. 40

Wagner, J.W. & de Groot, J. (1963) Effect of goldthioglucose injections on survival, organ damage and obesity in the rat. Proc. Soc. exp. Biol. (N.Y.), 112, 33-37

Waxler, S.H., Tabar, P. & Melcher, L.R. (1953) Obesity and the time of appearance of spontaneous mammary carcinoma in C3H mice. Cancer Res., 13, 276-278

1. Chemical and Physical Data

1.1 Synonyms and trade names

Chem. Abstr. Reg. Serial No.: 54-05-7

Chem. Abstr. Name: N^4-(7-Chloro-4-quinolinyl)-N^1,N^1-diethyl-1,4-pentanediamine

Chloraquine; 7-chloro-4-(4-diethylamino-1-methylbutylamino)quinoline; 7-chloro-4-{[4-(diethylamino)-1-methylbutyl]amino}quinoline; chloroquinium

Amokin; Aralen; Arechin; Arthrochin; Artrichin; Avlochlor; Avloclor; Bemaco; Bemaphate; Bemasulph; Benaquin; Bipiquin; Chemochin; Chingamin; Chlorochin; Chlorquin; Cidanchin; Clorochina; Chloroquina; Cocartrit; Delagil; Dichinalex; Elestol; Gontochin; Heliopar; Imagon; Iroquine; Klorokin; Lapaquin; Malaquin; Malaren; Malarex; Mesylith; Neochin; Nivachine; Nivaquine B; Quinachlor; Quinercyl; Quingamin; Quingamine; Quinilon; Quinoscan; Resochen; Resochin; Resoquina; Resoquine; Reumachlor; Reumaquin; Roquine; RP 3377; Sanoquin; Silbesan; Siragan; SN 6718; SN 7618; Solprina; Sopaquin; Tanakan; Tresochin; Trochin; W 7618; Win 244

1.2 Chemical formula and molecular weight

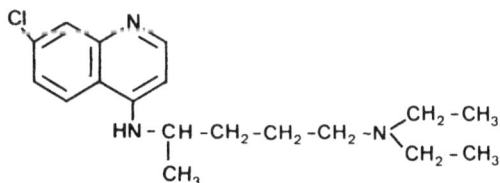

$C_{18}H_{26}ClN_3$ Mol. wt: 319.9

1.3 Chemical and physical properties of the pure substance

From US Pharmacopeial Convention, Inc. (1975), unless otherwise specified

(a) Description: White crystalline powder

(b) Melting-point: $87^{\circ}C$ (Stecher, 1968)

(c) Spectroscopy data: λ_{max} 220 nm (Viala et al., 1973), 255, 329 and 343 nm (WHO, 1967) in mineral acids

(d) Solubility: Very slightly soluble in water; soluble in dilute acids, chloroform and ether

1.4 Technical products and impurities

Various national and international pharmacopoeias give specifications for the purity of chloroquine and its salts in pharmaceutical products. For example, chloroquine is available in the US as a USP grade containing 98-102% active ingredient on a dried basis, as chloroquine hydrochloride injection, as chloroquine phosphate on a dried basis and in tablets (US Pharmacopeial Convention, Inc., 1975). Chloroquine phosphate and sulphate are available in the UK, containing no less than 98% active ingredient on a dried basis, for injection (95-100% of the stated amount) and in tablets (92.5-107.5% of the stated amount) (British Pharmacopoeia Commission, 1973). Combinations of chloroquine with other anti-malarial agents, e.g., pyrimethamine, are also available in some countries.

2. Production, Use, Occurrence and Analysis

For important background information on this section, see preamble, p. 15.

2.1 Production and use

(a) Production

Chloroquine was synthesized in Germany as early as 1934 (Rollo, 1975). It can be prepared by condensing 4,7-dichloroquinoline with 1-diethylamino-4-aminopentane (Harvey, 1975).

In the US, commercial production of chloroquine was first reported in 1949 (US Tariff Commission, 1950); however, it is usually manufactured as the phosphate or chloride salt. In 1974, only one US company reported production (see preamble, p. 15) of the phosphate salt (US International Trade Commission, 1976a). US imports of chloroquine phosphate were reported to have been about 100 kg in 1972 (US Tariff Commission, 1973), 500 kg in 1973 (US Tariff Commission, 1974) and 1300 kg in 1974 (US International Trade Commission, 1976b).

Production, importation and use of chloroquine in Japan are believed to have been minimal due to the risk of adverse effects involving optical retinopathy.

India was reported to have two producers of chloroquine, with a combined production of 23,820 kg in 1972. Indian imports were reported to be 99,330 kg for the period 1972-1973 (Anon., 1974).

(b) Use

Chloroquine was first developed and is currently used as an anti-malarial agent in human medicine. Partially immune adults infected with chloroquine-sensitive parasites may need only a single dose of 600 mg chloroquine to terminate a mild attack. Non-immune adults are given 1.5-2.4 g chloroquine or amodiaquine in divided doses over 3-5 days. Many dosage variations exist, but most are based on the administration of 900 mg chloroquine in divided doses on the first day, followed by smaller doses on subsequent days (WHO, 1973).

Combinations of chloroquine with other drugs, such as quinine, dapsone, pyrimethamine, sulphafurazole and sulphadiazine have been used against chloroquine-resistant *Plasmodium falciparum* malaria (WHO, 1973).

Chloroquine is also used as an efficient suppressive in all forms of malaria. The adult dose is either 300 mg chloroquine weekly or 100 mg daily on 6 days of each week depending on the transmission level in the area. Protective doses for children range from 37 mg chloroquine base for ages under one year to 225 mg chloroquine for ages 11-16 years, given weekly (Covell *et al.*, 1955).

As a lupus erythematosus suppressant, chloroquine is administered orally in two 150 mg doses daily for 1 to 2 weeks and then 150 mg daily thereafter (Harvey, 1975). It can also be employed in the treatment of extra-intestinal amoebiasis (Kastrup, 1971).

2.2 Occurrence

Chloroquine is not known to occur in nature.

2.3 Analysis

Methods for the estimation of chloroquine have been reviewed (Vykydal *et al.*, 1967). Those that meet regulatory requirements for pharmaceutical products include aqueous titration, non-aqueous titration and UV spectrophotometry. Determination of chloroquine in biological samples is most frequently carried out by spectrofluorimetric methods, although gas chromatography and colorimetric methods are also employed.

In spectrofluorimetric determinations, pH conditions for maximum sensitivity have been investigated (Schulman & Young, 1974). A comparison of three photochemical fluorimetric measuring techniques showed that digital integration of the fluorescence of chloroquine was the most sensitive, giving a limit of detection of 0.1 µg/1 (Lukasiewicz & Fitzgerald, 1974). Both spectrofluorimetric and UV spectrophotometric methods have been employed for determination of chloroquine after separation by thin-layer chromatography. The limits of detection by UV spectrophotometry were 0.17 µg/ml for blood, 0.05 µg/ml for urine and 1.07 µg/g for tissue; these values were about 9 times higher than the corresponding limits using spectrofluorimetry (Viala *et al.*, 1973).

Limits of detection for gas chromatography using flame ionization detection were 0.15 µg/ml for urine, 0.25 µg/ml for blood and 1.50 µg/g for tissue (Viala *et al.*, 1975).

A system of colorimetric tests for the presence of chloroquine in autopsy material, which is claimed to be specific, can detect 10 µg of the drug (Fartushnyi, 1967).

3. Biological Data Relevant to the Evaluation of Carcinogenic Risk to Man

3.1 Carcinogenicity and related studies in animals

Oral administration

Rat: Groups of 10 male and 10 female 21-day old Osborne-Mendel rats were given 0 (control), 100, 200, 400, 800 or 1000 mg chloroquine per kg of diet for up to 2 years. Inhibition of growth was severe at the 800 and 1000 mg/kg levels but temporary at 400 mg/kg. The toxicity of chloroquine became progressively more severe with increasing dosage, and 100% mortality was observed at the two highest dose levels at 35 and 25 weeks, respectively. No tumours were reported in 86 treated rats or in 15 control rats examined microscopically (Fitzhugh *et al.*, 1948; Nelson & Fitzhugh, 1948) [The Working Group noted the low number of survivors.]

3.2 Other relevant biological data

(a) Experimental systems

The oral LD_{50} of chloroquine phosphate is 620 mg/kg in mice, 970 mg/kg in rats and 136 mg/kg in rabbits (Sunshine, 1969). In a 2-year chronic toxicity study in rats fed diets containing from 100 to 1000 mg chloroquine/kg of diet, progressive retardation of growth and an increase in mortality were observed with levels of 800 and 1000 mg/kg of diet. Myocardial and voluntary muscle damage, centrilobular necrosis of the liver and testicular atrophy were also observed (Fitzhugh *et al.*, 1948).

Orally administered chloroquine is well and rapidly absorbed by many species (McChesney & McAuliff, 1961). It is deposited at up to 1000 times the plasma concentration in spleen, liver, kidney and lung and to a lesser degree in other tissues (McChesney *et al.*, 1967a). Extensive accumulation occurs in melanin-containing tissues (Lindquist, 1973; McChesney *et al.*, 1967a). In rats, up to 88% of extractable tissue-bound material was unchanged chloroquine (McChesney *et al.*, 1965); in monkeys, the main metabolite is 4-(7-chloroquinolyl)-γ-amino-*n*-valeric acid (Rollo, 1970). Chloroquine rapidly crosses the placenta in mice (Lindquist, 1973).

The drug interacts non-covalently with double-stranded DNA *in vitro* (Cohen & Yielding, 1965a; O'Brien *et al.*, 1966; Waring, 1970) and inhibits the activity of DNA polymerase (Cohen & Yielding, 1965b), DNA synthesis in mammalian cells (Cleaver & Painter, 1975) and DNA repair both in bacteria (Yielding *et al.*, 1970) and in mammalian cells (Michael & Williams, 1974).

(b) Man

High-dose, long-term therapy (more than one year) may result in retinopathy with doses exceeding 100 g (Voipio, 1966) and in ototoxicity (Hart & Naunton, 1964).

Chloroquine is well absorbed from the gastrointestinal tract and avidly retained in tissues. The main metabolite is de-ethylchloroquine (Rollo, 1975), but 70% is excreted as unchanged chloroquine (McChesney *et al.*, 1967b). When treatment with chloroquine alone or in combination with hydroxychloroquine is discontinued, chloroquine and its metabolites can be detected in the urine for up to 5 years (Rubin *et al.*, 1963).

3.3 Case reports and epidemiological studies

No data were available to the Working Group.

4. Comments on Data Reported and Evaluation

4.1 Animal data

The negative results obtained in the only available study in rats given chloroquine by oral administration did not form an adequate basis on which to make an evaluation of the carcinogenicity of this compound[1].

4.2 Human data

No case reports or epidemiological studies were available to the Working Group.

---

[1]The Working Group was aware of an on-going carcinogenicity study in mice (IARC, 1976).

52

5. References

Anon. (1974) Production and imports of selected drugs and pharmaceuticals in India. Chemical Industry News (India), July

British Pharmacopoeia Commission (1973) British Pharmacopoeia, London, HMSO, pp. 100-102

Cleaver, J.E. & Painter, R.B. (1975) Absence of specificity in inhibition of DNA repair replication by DNA-binding agents, cocarcinogens and steroids in human cells. Cancer Res., 35, 1773-1778

Cohen, S.N. & Yielding, K.L. (1965a) Spectrophotometric studies of the interaction of chloroquine with deoxyribonucleic acid. J. biol. Chem., 240, 3123-3131

Cohen, S.N. & Yielding, K.L. (1965b) Inhibition of DNA and RNA polymerase reactions by chloroquine. Proc. nat. Acad. Sci. (Wash.), 54, 521-527

Covell, G., Coatney, G.R., Field, J.W. & Singh, J. (1955) Chemotherapy of malaria. Wld Hlth Org. Monogr. Ser., No. 27, p. 87

Fartushnyi, A.F. (1967) Detecting chloroquine in autopsy matter. Sudebno-Med. Ekspertiza, Min. Zdravookhr. SSSR., 10, 45-48

Fitzhugh, O.G., Nelson, A.A. & Holland, O.L. (1948) The chronic oral toxicity of chloroquine. J. Pharmacol. exp. Ther., 93, 147-152

Hart, C.W. & Naunton, R.F. (1964) The ototoxicity of chloroquine phosphate. Arch. Otolaryngol., 80, 407-412

Harvey, S.C. (1975) Antimicrobial drugs. In: Osol, A. et al., eds, Remington's Pharmaceutical Sciences, 15th ed., Easton, Pa, Mack, pp. 1155-1156

IARC (1976) IARC Information Bulletin on the Survey of Chemicals Being Tested for Carcinogenicity, No. 6, Lyon, p. 233

Kastrup, E.K., ed. (1971) Facts and Comparisons, St Louis, Missouri, Facts and Comparisons, Inc., p. 378a

Lindquist, N.G. (1973) Accumulation of drugs on melanin. Acta radiol., Suppl. 325, 1-92

Lukasiewicz, R.J. & Fitzgerald, J.M. (1974) Comparison of three photo-chemical-fluorimetric methods for determination of chloroquine. Appl. Spectr., 28, 151-155

McChesney, E.W. & McAuliff, J.P. (1961) Laboratory studies of the 4-aminoquinoline antimalarials. I. Some biochemical characteristics of chloroquine, hydroxychloroquine, and SN-7718. Antibiot. Chemother., 11, 800-810

McChesney, E.W., Banks, W.F., Jr & Sullivan, D.J. (1965) Metabolism of chloroquine and hydroxychloroquine in albino and pigmented rats. Toxicol. appl. Pharmacol., 7, 627-636

McChesney, E.W., Banks, W.F., Jr & Fabian, R.J. (1967a) Tissue distribution of chloroquine, hydroxychloroquine and desethylchloroquine in the rat. Toxicol. appl. Pharmacol., 10, 501-513

McChesney, E.W., Fasco, M.J. & Banks, W.F., Jr (1967b) The metabolism of chloroquine in man during and after repeated oral dosage. J. Pharmacol. exp. Ther., 158, 323-331

Michael, R.O. & Williams, G.M. (1974) Chloroquine inhibition of repair of DNA damage induced in mammalian cells by methyl methanesulfonate. Mutation Res., 25, 391-396

Nelson, A.A. & Fitzhugh, O.G. (1948) Chloroquine (SN-7618). Pathologic changes observed in rats which for two years had been fed various proportions. Arch. Path., 45, 454-462

O'Brien, R.L., Allison, J.L. & Hahn, F.E. (1966) Evidence for intercalation of chloroquine into DNA. Biochim. biophys. acta, 129, 622-624

Rollo, I.M. (1970) Drugs used in the chemotherapy of malaria. In: Goodman, L.S. & Gilman, A., eds, The Pharmacological Basis of Therapeutics, 4th ed., New York, Macmillan, pp. 1101-1105

Rollo, I.M. (1975) Drugs used in the chemotherapy of malaria. In: Goodman, L.S. & Gilman, A., eds, The Pharmacological Basis of Therapeutics, 5th ed., New York, Macmillan, pp. 1049-1053

Rubin, M., Bernstein, H.N. & Zvaifler, N.J. (1963) Studies on the pharmacology of chloroquine: recommendations for the treatment of chloroquine retinopathy. Arch. Ophthamol., 70, 474-481

Schulman, S.G. & Young, J.F. (1974) A modified fluorimetric determination of chloroquine in biological samples. Analyt. chim. acta, 70, 229-232

Stecher, P.G., ed. (1968) The Merck Index, 8th ed., Rahway, NJ, Merck & Co., p. 247

Sunshine, I., ed. (1969) CRC Handbook of Analytical Toxicology, Cleveland, Ohio, Chemical Rubber Co., p. 29

US International Trade Commission (1976a) Synthetic Organic Chemicals, US Production and Sales, 1974, USITC Publication 776, Washington DC, US Government Printing Office, p. 101

US International Trade Commission (1976b) Imports of Benzenoid Chemicals and Products, 1974, USITC Publication 762, Washington DC, US Government Printing Office, p. 81

US Pharmacopeial Convention, Inc. (1975) The US Pharmacopeia, 19th rev., RockvilMd, pp. 81-83

US Tariff Commission (1950) Synthetic Organic Chemicals, US Production and Sales, 1949, Report No. 169, Second Series, Washington DC, US Government Printing Office, p. 101

US Tariff Commission (1973) Imports of Benzenoid Chemicals and Products, 1972, TC Publication 601, Washington DC, US Government Printing Office, p. 83

US Tariff Commission (1974) Imports of Benzenoid Chemicals and Products, 1973, TC Publication 688, Washington DC, US Government Printing Office, p. 79

Viala, A., Gouezo, F. & Durand, A. (1973) Dosage de la chloroquine et évaluation de ses métabolites dans les milieux biologiques par spectro-fluorimetrie. Trav. Soc. pharm. Montpellier, 33, 389-397

Viala, A., Cano, J.P. & Durand, A. (1975) Dosage de la chloroquine dans les milieux biologiques par chromatographie en phase gazeuse. J. Chromat., 111, 299-303

Voipio, H. (1966) Incidence of chloroquine retinopathy. Acta ophthal. (Kbh), 44, 349-354

Vykydal, M., Pegrimova, E., Demkova, V. & Kalab, M. (1967) Estimation of chloroquine in the organism. Cas. Lek. Cesk., 106, 44-47

Waring, M. (1970) Variation of the supercoils in closed circular DNA by binding of antibiotics and drugs: evidence for molecular models involving intercalation. J. mol. Biol., 54, 247-279

WHO (1967) Specifications for the Quality Controls of Pharmaceutical Preparations, Second Edition of the International Pharmacopoeia, Geneva, pp. 116-119, 621

WHO (1973) Chemotherapy of malaria and resistance to antimalarials. Wld Hlth Org. techn. Rep. Ser., No. 529, pp. 7, 19-23

Yielding, K.L., Yielding, L. & Gaudin, D. (1970) Inhibition by chloroquine of UV repair in E. coli B[1]. Proc. Soc. exp. Biol. (N.Y.), 133, 999-1001

1. Chemical and Physical Data

Diazepam

1.1 Synonyms and trade names

Chem. Abstr. Reg. Serial No.: 439-14-5

Chem. Abstr. Name: 7-Chloro-1,3-dihydro-1-methyl-5-phenyl-2H-1,4-benzodiazepin-2-one

7-Chloro-1-methyl-5-3H-1,4-benzodiazepin-2(1H)-one; 7-chloro-1-methyl-2-oxo-5-phenyl-3H-1,4-benzodiazepine; 7-chloro-1-methyl-5-phenyl-2H-1,4-benzodiazepin-2-one; 7-chloro-1-methyl-5-phenyl-3H-1,4-benzodiazepin-2(1H)-one; 7-chloro-1-methyl-5-phenyl-1,3-dihydro-2H-1,4-benzodiazepin-2-one; diacepan; diazepan; methyldiazepinone; 1-methyl-5-phenyl-7-chloro-1,3-dihydro-2H-1,4-benzodiazepin-2-one

Alboral; Aliseum; Amiprol; Ansiolin; Ansiolisina; Apaurin; Apozepam; Assival; Atensine; Atilen; Bialzepam; Calmocitene; Calmpose; Cercine; Ceregulart; Condition; Diapam; Diazetard; Dienpax; Dipam; Dipezona; Domalium; Duksen; Duxen; E-Pam; Eridan; Faustan; Freudal; Gihitan; Horizon; Kiatrium; LA III; Lembrol; Levium; Liberetas; Morosan; Noan; Pacitran; Paranten; Paxate; Paxel; Plidan; Quetinil; Quiatril; Quievita; Relanium; Relax; Renborin; Ro 5-2807; S.A. R.L.; Saromet; Sedipam; Seduxen; Serenack; Serenamin; Serenzin; Setonil; Sonacon; Stesolid; Stesolin; Tensopam; Tranimul; Tranqdyn; Tranquirit; Umbrium; Unisedil; Usempax AP; Valeo; Valitran; Valium; Vatran; Velium; Vival; Vivol; Wy 3467; Zipan

1.2 Chemical formula and molecular weight

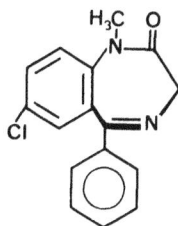

$C_{16}H_{13}ClN_2O$

Mol. wt: 284.8

1.3 Chemical and physical properties of the pure substance

From Stecher (1968), unless otherwise specified

(a) Description: Plates

(b) Melting-point: 125-126°C

(c) Spectroscopy data: λ_{max} 242, 285 and 368 nm in acidified ethanol; infra-red, nuclear magnetic resonance and mass spectra have been reported (MacDonald et al., 1972).

(d) Solubility: Slightly soluble in water; soluble in ethanol; freely soluble in chloroform (US Pharmacopeial Convention, Inc., 1975)

1.4 Technical products and impurities

Various national and international pharmacopoeias give specifications for the purity of diazepam in pharmaceutical products. For example, diazepam is available in the US as a National Formulary or USP grade containing 98.5-101.0% active ingredient on a dried basis with a maximum of 0.002% heavy metals. Injections of a sterile solution of diazepam in water or other suitable media [such as solutions of propylene glycol, ethanol, sodium benzoate, benzoic acid or benzyl alcohol (Kastrup, 1976)] are available in a dose of 5 mg diazepam per ml containing 90-110% of the stated amount. Diazepam tablets are also available in 2, 5 and 10 mg doses containing 90.0-110.0% of the stated amount of diazepam (National Formulary Board, 1970; US Pharmacopeial Convention, Inc., 1975). In Japan, diazepam is also available in powders and capsules. In the UK, diazepam is available on a dried basis, containing 99-101% active ingredient, and in capsules and tablets containing 92.5-107.5% of the stated amount (British Pharmacopoeia Commission, 1973).

Oxazepam

1.1 Synonyms and trade names

Chem. Abstr. Reg. Serial No.: 604-75-1

Chem. Abstr. Name: 7-Chloro-1,3-dihydro-3-hydroxy-5-phenyl-2H-1,4-benzodiazepin-2-one

7-Chloro-1,3-dihydro-3-hydroxy-5-phenyl-2H-1,4-benzodiazepin-2-one;
7-chloro-3-hydroxy-5-phenyl-2H-1,4-benzodiazepin-2-one; 7-chloro-3-
hydroxy-5-phenyl-1,3-dihydro-2H-1,4-benzodiazepin-2-one

Adumbran; Ansioxacepam; Anxiolit; Aplakil; Astress; Bonare;
Enidrel; Isodin; Limbial; Nesontil; Praxiten; Propax; Psicopax;
Quen; Quilibrex; Ro 5-6789; Rondar; Serax; Serenal; Serenid;
Serenid-D; Serepax; Seresta; Serpax; Tazepam; Vaben; Wy-3498;
Z 10 TR

1.2 Chemical formula and molecular weight

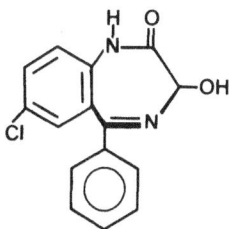

$C_{15}H_{11}ClN_2O_2$

Mol. wt: 286.7

1.3 Chemical and physical properties of the pure substance

From Stecher (1968), unless otherwise specified

(a) Description: Crystals from ethanol

(b) Melting-point: 205-206°C

(c) Spectroscopy data: λ_{max} 230 and 318 nm in ethanol; 236, 284
and 362 nm in 0.1 N hydrochloric acid; infra-red, nuclear
magnetic resonance and mass spectra have been reported
(Shearer & Pilla, 1974).

(d) Solubility: Soluble in ethanol (0.45 g/100 ml), chloroform
(0.4 g/100 ml) and dioxane; practically insoluble in water
(0.003 g/100 ml) (Shearer & Pilla, 1974)

(e) Stability: Stable as a solid or in neutral solutions but
hydrolysed by acids (Shearer & Pilla, 1974)

1.4 Technical products and impurities

Oxazepam is available in the US as a National Formulary grade containing
98-102% active ingredient on a dried basis. Capsules are available in
10, 15 and 30 mg doses containing 90-110% of the stated amount of
oxazepam (National Formulary Board, 1970). Tablets are also available,
in 15 mg doses (Kastrup, 1974). Oxazepam is available in Japan in powder
form.

2. Production, Use, Occurrence and Analysis

For important background information on this section, see preamble,
p. 15.

2.1 Production and use

(a) Production

A method of preparing diazepam was first reported in 1961; benzoyl
chloride is reacted with *para*-chloroaniline in the presence of a zinc
chloride catalyst. The resulting 2-amino-5-chlorobenzophenone is converted
to the oxime with hydroxylamine and then cyclized to the chloromethyl-
quinazoline-3-oxide by treatment with chloroacetyl chloride. When this
is treated with alkali, ring enlargement occurs, giving 7-chloro-1,3-
dihydro-5-phenyl-2H-1,4-benzodiazepin-2-one-4-oxide. Raney nickel reduction
of the oxide followed by methylation with dimethyl sulphate gives diazepam
(Sternbach & Reeder, 1961; Sternbach *et al.*, 1961). Diazepam has also
been prepared by the reaction of 2-methylamino-5-chlorobenzophenone with
ethyl glycinate (Reeder & Sternbach, 1963), or with bromoacetyl bromide
followed by reaction with ammonia (Reeder & Sternbach, 1964).

Preparation of oxazepam was first reported in 1962; in this method
6-chloro-2-chloromethyl-4-phenylquinazoline 3-oxide is treated with sodium
hydroxide to give 7-chloro-5-phenyl-1,3-dihydro-2H-1,4-benzodiazepin-2-
one-4-oxide. This rearranges to the 3-acetyloxy derivative when treated
with acetic anhydride. Reaction of this with sodium hydroxide forms a
precipitate, which, after dissolution in water and acidification with
acetic acid, gives oxazepam (Bell & Childress, 1962).

Commercial production of diazepam was first reported in the US in 1963
(US Tariff Commission, 1964); only one US company reported production (see
preamble, p. 15) in 1974 (US International Trade Commission, 1976a). US
imports of diazepam through the principal customs districts were 33 kg
in 1974 (US International Trade Commission, 1976b).

Commercial production of oxazepam was first reported in the US in
1965 (US Tariff Commission, 1967); only one US company reported production
(see preamble, p. 15) in 1974 (US International Trade Commission, 1976a).
US imports of oxazepam through the principal customs districts were
560 kg in 1973 (US Tariff Commission, 1974).

No evidence was found that diazepam or oxazepam is produced commercially
in Japan. In 1975, Japan imported 135 kg diazepam, principally from
Argentina, with smaller amounts from Denmark and Canada, and over 200 kg
oxazepam, principally from Turkey.

Annual production of diazepam is less than 1,000 kg in each of the
following countries: Austria, Benelux, France, Scandinavia and the UK;
1-100 thousand kg are produced in the Federal Republic of Germany, in Italy,
in Spain and in Switzerland. Annual production of oxazepam is less than
1,000 kg in Austria, in Benelux, in the Federal Republic of Germany, in
France, in Scandinavia, in Spain, in Switzerland and in the UK; 1-100
thousand kg are produced in Italy. Annual production of both diazepam and
oxazepam in eastern Europe is estimated to be in the range of 1-100
thousand kg.

(b) Use

Diazepam is widely used for the treatment of anxiety in a usual dose
range of 5-20 mg/day. It has also been used as a skeletal muscle relaxant
in various spastic disorders (2-20 mg intravenously at intervals of 2-8
hours), as a pre-anaesthetic medication in childbirth and cardioversion
(i.v. doses of 5-30 mg) and as a hypnotic antiepileptic agent (Byck, 1975).
The usual route of administration for treatment of chronic diseases is oral,
but an injectable solution of 5 mg/ml is available for acute disorders
(Woodbury & Fingl, 1975).

Oxazepam, a metabolite of diazepam, is primarily used in human medicine for the treatment of anxiety and tension (Grollman & Grollman, 1970); it has also been used as an antiepileptic agent (Woodbury & Fingl, 1975). The usual dose range is 30-90 mg/day given in capsules of 10 to 30 mg (Byck, 1975).

Because of potential abuse of both diazepam and oxazepam, leading to limited physical or psychological dependence on these drugs, on 1 April 1976, the US Drug Enforcement Agency placed diazepam and oxazepam in Schedule IV of the Controlled Substances Act, which requires all manufacturers and distributors of these compounds to register and report to the agency any changes in the quantity manufactured and distributed and requires physicians to review their patients' status periodically (US Drug Enforcement Administration, 1975, 1976).

It has been reported that about three billion tablets of diazepam were sold in the US in 1974 (Anon., 1975). Total US sales of oxazepam for use in human medicine are estimated to be less than 3,000 kg annually.

2.2 Occurrence

Neither diazepam nor oxazepam is known to occur in nature.

2.3 Analysis

Compilations of analytical methods for the determination of diazepam (MacDonald *et al.*, 1972) and of oxazepam (Shearer & Pilla, 1974) have been published. Methods of assaying diazepam that meet regulatory requirements for pharmaceutical products include non-aqueous titration and UV spectrophotometry.

A method using thin-layer chromatography prior to spectrophotometric analysis can separate diazepam in pharmaceutical formulations from its degradation product (Sbarbati Nudelman & De Waisbaum, 1975). A two-dimensional thin-layer chromatographic method can separate and detect five similar tranquilizer drugs (including diazepam) (Schuetz *et al.*, 1972).

A gravimetric and complexometric method for the determination of diazepam is based on the formation of the hexathiocyanatochromate (III) (Grecu & Marcu, 1973).

A colorimetric method has been developed to determine diazepam as the pure drug and in formulations by hydrolysis in chloroform to 2-methylamino-5-chlorobenzophenone, a deep-yellow compound (Baggi *et al.*, 1975). Another colorimetric method, developed for the detection of primary amines on thin-layer plates, was found to be applicable to diazepam, apparently because diazepam decomposes on the plate (Haefelfinger, 1970).

A polarographic method allows simultaneous determination of three 1,4-benzodiazepine drugs (including diazepam) (Oelschlaeger & Volke, 1966). A rapid-pulse polarographic method to determine diazepam in serum has a detection limit of 0.01 µg/ml (Jacobsen *et al.*, 1973).

One gas-liquid chromatographic method uses electron capture detection capable of detecting the metabolites of medazepam (such as diazepam) in blood and urine at the 0.04-0.05 µg/ml level; the method involves hydrolysis to the benzophenone derivatives (de Silva & Puglisi, 1970). A similar method for its detection in serum using flame ionization detection has been described (Steyn & Hundt, 1975). A gas chromatographic method can determine diazepam and its major metabolites in biological materials quantitatively, with a limit of detection of 0.003 µg/ml (Heidbrink *et al.*, 1975). Gas chromatographic-mass spectrometric methods are used to determine diazepam and its metabolites in biological materials (Horning *et al.*, 1974) and to analyse the stability of bulk diazepam at gas chromatograph temperatures (Sadée & van der Kleijn, 1971). A high-pressure liquid chromatographic method separates and determines diazepam at the microgram level (Scott & Bommer, 1970).

Oxazepam can be assayed by gravimetric analysis using silicotungstic acid (Baltazar & Ferreira Braga, 1967); non-aqueous titrimetric methods can be used to determine bulk oxazepam (Baltazar & Ferreira Braga, 1967; Beyer & Sadée, 1967; National Formulary Board, 1970; Salim *et al.*, 1968), and UV spectrophotometry can be used to determine oxazepam in capsules (National Formulary Board, 1970; Salim *et al.*, 1968).

Oxazepam and its metabolites can be assayed colorimetrically in biological materials by hydrolsis to 2-amino-5-chlorobenzophenone and diazotizing and coupling with α-naphthol (Pelzer & Maass, 1969), *N-α-*

naphthyl-N'-diethyl propylenediamine (Lafargue *et al.*, 1970) or N-(1-naphthyl)ethylenediamine hydrochloride (Kamm & Kelm, 1969).

A fluorimetric method can determine oxazepam in biological fluids (Walkenstein *et al.*, 1964). Polarographic methods are used to analyse bulk oxazepam in a methanol-methylene chloride solvent system (Fazzari & Riggleman, 1969) and to analyse oxazepam tablets in Britton-Robinson buffer solutions containing 20% dimethylformamide (Oelschlaeger *et al.*, 1969).

Gas chromatographic-mass spectrometric methods to analyse oxazepam, in which oxazepam is quantitatively rearranged to the quinazoline carbox-aldehyde (Sadée & van der Kleijn, 1971), and to determine the metabolite of oxazepam, oxazepam glucuronide, in urine (Marcucci *et al.*, 1975) have been developed.

A high-pressure liquid chromatographic procedure to separate mixtures of pure benzodiazepines (including oxazepam) has been described (Scott & Bommer, 1970).

3. Biological Data Relevant to the Evaluation of Carcinogenic Risk to Man

3.1 Carcinogenicity and related studies in animals

Oral administration

Mouse: Three groups of 14 male and 14 female Swiss-Webster mice received oxazepam in the diet from 3 to 12 months of age at concentrations of 0.05 or 0.15%, or were given a control diet. At 12 months of age all mice received the control diet for a further 2 months; then, all surviving animals were killed. Liver tumours described as liver-cell adenomas were found in 3/12 (25%) males receiving the lower dose and in 8/13 (61%) males and 5/8 (62%) females receiving 0.15% oxazepam. No liver tumours were seen in 13 male and 10 female surviving controls (Fox & Lahcen, 1974).

3.2 Other relevant biological data

(a) Experimental systems

The oral LD_{50} of diazepam in mice is 278 mg/kg bw and that of oxazepam, 1540 mg/kg bw (Marcucci *et al.*, 1968).

N_1-Demethylation and C_3-hydroxylation of diazepam lead to formation of *N*-demethyldiazepam, 3-hydroxydiazepam and oxazepam, which are excreted as glucuronides in mice (Marcucci *et al.*, 1968), rats (Schwartz *et al.*, 1967), guinea-pigs (Marcucci *et al.*, 1971), rabbits (Jommi *et al.*, 1964) and dogs (Ruelius *et al.*, 1965; Schwartz *et al.*, 1965). In addition, *para*-hydroxylation of the 5-phenyl ring occurs in rats (Schwartz *et al.*, 1967) and rabbits (Jommi *et al.*, 1964).

Oxazepam has also been identified as a metabolite of chlordiazepoxide (librium) in dogs (Kimmel & Walkenstein, 1967). Orally administered oxazepam is metabolized to 6-chloro-4-phenyl-2-(1*H*)-quinazolinone, 5-*para*-hydroxyoxazepam and the three open-ring metabolites (free or conjugated), 2-amino-5-chlorobenzophenone, 2'-benzoyl-4'-chloro-2,2-dihydroxy-acetanilide and 2'-benzoyl-4'-chloro-2-hydroxy-2-ureidoacetanilide, in miniature swine (Sisenwine *et al.*, 1972).

In vitro studies showed that liver of dogs (Schwartz & Postma, 1968), rats and mice (Kvetina *et al.*, 1968) metabolizes diazepam to form the three metabolic products, *N*-demethyldiazepam, 3-hydroxydiazepam and oxazepam.

By whole body autoradiography, rapid and intense accumulation of ^{14}C-labelled diazepam was observed in brain, kidney, liver, myocardium and body fat of mice (van der Kleijn, 1969) and of newborn rhesus monkeys (van der Kleijn & Wijffels, 1971). Following i.v. administration of diazepam it was found that *N*-demethyldiazepam accumulated in the blood and brain of mice (Marcucci *et al.*, 1968), in blood, brain and adipose tissue of quinea-pigs (Marcucci *et al.*, 1971) and in very small amounts for a short time in the blood, brain and adipose tissue of rats (Marcucci *et al.*, 1970).

Dogs given diazepam intravenously excrete 61% of the compound and its metabolites in the urine and 34% in the faeces (Schwartz *et al.*, 1965). Transplacental transfer of diazepam occurred in mice, hamsters and monkeys (Idänpään-Heikkilä *et al.*, 1971a,b).

When pregnant A/J mice were given a single i.m. dose of 100 mg/kg bw diazepam on the 14th day of pregnancy, no changes in the incidence of cleft palate were observed in the offspring (Walker & Patterson, 1974).

Oxazepam did not cause non-disjunction and crossing-over in *Aspergillus nidulans* (Bignami *et al.*, 1974); mammalian metabolic activating systems were not used in this test.

(b) Man

The major metabolites of diazepam in humans are formed by N-demethylation and C$_3$-hydroxylation (Schwartz *et al.*, 1965). The main blood metabolite, *N*-demethyldiazepam (Kaplan *et al.*, 1973), appears in the plasma within 1-1.5 hours after i.m. administration (Baird & Hailey, 1973). Diazepam metabolites are almost completely conjugated before excretion; oxazepam-glucuronide is a major urinary metabolite. Schwartz *et al.* (1965) found 10% *N*-demethyldiazepam, 10% 3-hydroxydiazepam, and somewhat more than 30% oxazepam in the urine; approximately 71% of orally administered diazepam and its metabolites are excreted in the urine and 10% in the faeces.

Oxazepam is metabolized to 6-chloro-4-phenyl-2(1*H*)-quinazolinone, 5-*para*-hydroxyoxazepam and the 3 open-ring metabolites, 2-amino-5-chlorobenzo-phenone, 2'-benzoyl-4'-chloro-2,2-dihydroxyacetanilide and 2'-benzoyl-4'-chloro-2-hydroxy-2-ureidoacetanilide in humans (Sisenwine *et al.*, 1972).

Diazepam and its metabolite *N*-demethyldiazepam cross the placenta readily when diazepam is given to mothers during labour (Erkkola *et al.*, 1973) or at the end of the first trimester of pregnancy (Erkkola *et al.*, 1974; Idänpään-Heikkilä *et al.*, 1971c). The tissue concentration of diazepam in the foetus was higher than that in the mother; the concentration of *N*-demethyldiazepam in foetal liver was exceptionally high (Errkola *et al.*, 1974).

A significant association was found between maternal intake of diazepam during the first trimester of pregnancy and the frequency of oral clefts in the children. Of 709 women interviewed, 21 reported first-trimester exposure to diazepam. A computer screen identified a statistically signifi-cant four-fold relative risk for first-trimester exposure to diazepam among the mothers of infants with cleft lip with or without cleft palate as compared with the mothers of infants with all other defects. Similar results were obtained using mongolism as the control, but the significance levels were lower due to smaller sample size. In no other defect category did first-trimester use of diazepam differ significantly from that of the rest of the group (Safra & Oakley, 1975).

In the years 1967-71 information was collected on the mothers of 599 children with oral clefts; for 590 matched pair controls the data were considered adequate. The material was divided into three groups - cleft palate (CP), cleft lip with or without cleft palate (CL±CP) and clefts with additional defects. When the anti-anxiety drugs were divided into two groups - benzodiazepines (diazepam, oxazepam, nitrazepam, chlordiazepoxide) and 'other' (meprobamate, chlormezanone) - a significant association was found (P<0.05) between intake of benzodiazepines during the first trimester of pregnancy and oral clefts: the association was significant in the CP group; an increased intake of these drugs was also seen in the CL±CP group when compared to controls, but the difference was not significant (Saxén & Saxén, 1975).

3.3 Case reports and epidemiological studies

No data were available to the Working Group.

4. Comments on Data Reported and Evaluation[1]

4.1 Animal data

In the only report available, oxazepam, a major metabolite of diazepam, was carcinogenic in mice after its oral administration: it produced liver-cell tumours.

4.2 Human data

No case reports or epidemiological studies were available to the Working Group.

---

[1]See also the section 'Animal Data in Relation to the Evaluation of Risk to Man' in the introduction to this volume, p. 13.

5. References

Anon. (1975) Librium and valium. *Drug and Cosmetic Industry*, July, p. 85

Baggi, T.R., Mahajan, S.N. & Rao, G.R. (1975) Colorimetric determination of diazepam in pharmaceutical preparations. *J. Ass. off. analyt. Chem.*, 58, 875-878

Baird, E.S. & Hailey, D.M. (1973) Plasma levels of diazepam and its major metabolite following intramuscular administration. *Brit. J. Anaes.*, 45, 546-548

Baltazar, J. & Ferreira Braga, M.M. (1967) Some physico-chemical characteristics and dosage methods of oxazepam. *Rev. Port. Farm.*, 17, 109-114

Bell, S.C. & Childress, S.J. (1962) A rearrangement of 5-aryl-1,3-dihydro-2*H*-1,4-benzodiazepine-2-one 4-oxides. *J. org. Chem.*, 27, 1691-1695

Beyer, K.H. & Sadée, W. (1967) Chemistry and analysis of benzodiazepine derivatives. III. Titration of benzodiazepine derivatives in anhydrous medium. *Arch. Pharm. (Weinheim)*, 300, 667-673

Bignami, M., Morpurgo, G., Pagliani, R., Carere, A., Conti, G. & Di Giuseppe, G. (1974) Non-disjunction and crossing-over induced by pharmaceutical drugs in *Aspergillus nidulans*. *Mutation Res.*, 26, 159-170

British Pharmacopoeia Commission (1973) *British Pharmacopoeia*, London, HMSO, pp. 154-155

Byck, R. (1975) *Drugs and the treatment of psychiatric disorders*. In: Goodman, L.S. & Gilman, A., eds, *The Pharmacological Basis of Therapeutics* 5th ed., New York, Macmillan, pp. 189-192

Erkkola, R., Kangas, L. & Pekkarinen, A. (1973) The transfer of diazepam across the placenta during labour. *Acta obstet. gynec. scand.*, 52, 167-170

Erkkola, R., Kanto, J. & Sellman, R. (1974) Diazepam in early human pregnancy. *Acta obstet. gynec. scand.*, 53, 135-138

Fazzari, F.R. & Riggleman, O.H. (1969) Polarographic determination of oxazepam. *J. pharm. Sci.*, 58, 1530-1531

Fox, K.A. & Lahcen, R.B. (1974) Liver-cell adenomas and peliosis hepatis in mice associated with oxazepam. *Res. Comm. chem. Path. Pharmacol.*, 8, 481-488

Grecu, I. & Marcu, P. (1973) Anionic complexes of Cr(III) in the analysis and the control of drugs. Applications, to the gravimetric and volumetric dosage of diazepam (valium, Ro-5-2807, WY 3467). Farmacia (Buc.), 21, 585-589

Grollman, A. & Grollman, E.F. (1970) Pharmacology and Therapeutics, 7th ed., Philadelphia, Lea & Febiger, p. 236

Haefelfinger, P. (1970) Empfindlicher Nachweis von Substanzen mit primären Aminogruppen auf Dünnschichtplatten. J. Chromat., 48, 184-190

Heidbrink, V., Mallach, H.J. & Moosmayer, A. (1975) Zur gaschromatographischen Analytik der Benzodiazepine. II. Diazepam und seine Metabolite. Arzneimittel-Forsch., 25, 516-517

Horning, M.G., Stillwell, W.G., Nowlin, J., Lertratanangkoon, K., Carroll, D., Dzidic, I., Stillwell, R.N. & Horning, E.C. (1974) The use of stable isotopes in gas chromatography-mass spectrometric studies of drug metabolism. J. Chromat., 91, 413-423

Idänpään-Heikkilä, J.E., Taska, R.J., Allen, H.A. & Schoolar, J.C. (1971a) Placental transfer of diazepam-^{14}C in mice, hamsters and monkeys. J. Pharmacol. exp. Ther., 176, 752-757

Idänpään-Heikkilä, J.E., Taska, R.J., Allen, H.A. & Schoolar, J.C. (1971b) Autoradiographic study of the fate of diazepam-C^{14} in the monkey brain. Arch. int. Pharmacodyn., 194, 68-77

Idänpään-Heikkilä, J.E., Jouppila, P.I., Puolakka, J.O. & Vorne, M.S. (1971c) Placental transfer and fetal metabolism of diazepam in early human pregnancy. Amer. J. Obstet. Gynec., 109, 1011-1016

Jacobsen, E., Jacobsen, T.V. & Rojahn, T. (1973) Determination of diazepam in serum by differential pulse polarography. Analyt. chim. acta, 64, 473-476

Jommi, G., Manitto, P. & Silanos, M.A. (1964) Metabolism of diazepam in rabbits. Arch. Biochem. Biophys., 108, 334-340

Kamm, G. & Kelm, R. (1969) Quantitativer Nachweis von 7-Chlor-1,3-dihydro-3-hydroxy-5-phenyl-2H-1,4-benzodiazepin-2-on im Plasma bei einmaliger und längerer Verabreichung. Arzneimittel-Forsch., 19, 1659-1662

Kaplan, S.A., Jack, M.L., Alexander, K. & Weinfeld, R.E. (1973) Pharmacokinetic profile of diazepam in man following single intravenous and oral and chronic oral administrations. J. pharm. Sci., 62, 1789-1796

Kastrup, E.K., ed. (1974) Facts and Comparisons, St Louis, Missouri, Facts and Comparisons, Inc., p. 261c

Kastrup, E.K., ed. (1976) Facts and Comparisons, St Louis, Missouri, Facts and Comparisons, Inc., p. 288f

Kimmel, H.B. & Walkenstein, S.S. (1967) Oxazepam excretion by chlordiaze-poxide-^{14}C-dosed dogs. J. pharm. Sci., 56, 538-539

van der Kleijn, E. (1969) Kinetics of distribution and metabolism of diazepam and chlordiazepoxide in mice. Arch. int. Pharmacodyn., 178, 193-215

van der Kleijn, E. & Wijffels, C.C.G. (1971) Whole-body and regional brain distribution of diazepam in newborn rhesus monkeys. Arch. int. Pharma-codyn., 192, 255-264

Kvetina, J., Marcucci, F. & Fanelli, R. (1968) Metabolism of diazepam in isolated perfused liver of rat and mouse. J. Pharm. Pharmacol., 20, 807-808

Lafargue, P., Pont, P. & Meunier, J. (1970) Etude des dérivés de la benzo-[f]-diazépine-1,4 utilisés en thérapeutique. I. Etude spéctroscopique et par chromatographie en couche mince de ces dérivés, de leurs principaux métabolites et des composés formés par leur hydrolyse acide. Ann. pharm. franç., 28, 343-354

MacDonald, A., Michaelis, A.F. & Senkowski, B.Z. (1972) Diazepam. In: Florey, K., ed., Analytical Profiles of Drug Substances, Vol. 1, New York, Academic Press, pp. 80-99

Marcucci, F., Guaitani, A., Kvetina, J., Mussini, E. & Garattini, S. (1968) Species difference in diazepam metabolism and anticonvulsant effect. Europ. J. Pharmacol., 4, 467-470

Marcucci, F., Fanelli, R., Mussini, E. & Garattini, S. (1970) Further studies on species difference in diazepam metabolism. Europ. J. Pharmacol., 9, 253-256

Marcucci, F., Guaitani, A., Fanelli, R., Mussini, E. & Garattini, S. (1971) Metabolism and anticonvulsant activity of diazepam in guinea-pigs. Biochem. Pharmacol., 20, 1711-1713

Marcucci, F., Bianchi, R., Airoldi, L., Salmona, M., Fanelli, R., Chiabrando, C., Frigerio, A., Mussini, E. & Garattini, S. (1975) Gas chromato-graphic-mass spectrometric determination of intact C_3-hydroxylated benzodiazepine glucuronides in urine. J. Chromat., 107, 285-293

National Formulary Board (1970) National Formulary XIII, Washington DC, American Pharmaceutical Association, pp. 220-223, 501-502

Oelschlaeger, H. & Volke, J. (1966) Polarography of therapeutically impor-tant 1,4-benzodiazepine derivatives. In: Hanc, O., ed., Proceedings of the 25th International Pharmaceutical Congress, 1966, Vol. 2, London, Butterworths, pp. 101-104

Oelschlaeger, H., Volke, J., Lim, G.T. & Spang, R. (1969) Pharmaceutical analysis by polarography and oscillopolarography. X. Reduction of oxazepam at the dropping mercury electrode. Arch. Pharm. (Weinheim), 302, 946-951

Pelzer, H. & Maass, D. (1969) Pharmakokinetik und Metabolismus von 7-Chlor-1,3-dihydro-3-hydroxy-5-phenyl-2H-1,4-benzodiazepin-2-on und dessen Hemisuccinat beim Menschen. Arzneimittel-Forsch., 19, 1652-1656

Reeder, E. & Sternbach, L.H. (1963) 5-Phenyl-1,2-dihydro-3H-1,4-benzo-diazepines. US Patent 3,109,843, November 5, to Hoffmann-La Roche Inc.

Reeder, E. & Sternbach, L.H. (1964) 5-Aryl-3H-1,4-benzodiazepin-2(1H)-ones. US Patent 3,136,815, June 9, to Hoffmann-La Roche Inc.

Ruelius, H.W., Lee, J.M. & Alburn, H.E. (1965) Metabolism of diazepam in dogs: transformation to oxazepam. Arch. Biochem. Biophys., 111, 376-380

Sadée, W. & van der Kleijn, E. (1971) Thermolysis of 1,4-benzodiazepines during gas chromatography and mass spectroscopy. J. pharm. Sci., 60, 135-137

Safra, M.J. & Oakley, G.P., Jr (1975) Association between cleft lip with or without cleft palate and prenatal exposure to diazepam. Lancet, ii, 478-480

Salim, E.F., Deuble, J.L. & Papariello, G. (1968) Qualitative and quantitative tests for oxazepam. J. pharm. Sci., 57, 311-313

Saxén, I. & Saxén, L. (1975) Association between maternal intake of diazepam and oral clefts. Lancet, ii, 498

Sbarbati Nudelman, N. & De Waisbaum, R.G. (1975) Method to determine diazepam and nitrazepam stability. Farmaco, Ed. prat., 30, 488-495

Schuetz, C., Post, D., Schewe, G., Schuetz, H. & Muskat, E. (1972) Microchemical detection and separation of five 5-phenyl-1,4-benzodiazepine tranquilizers by thin-layer chromatographical SRS-technique. Fresenius' Z. analyt. Chem., 262, 282-286

Schwartz, M.A. & Postma, E. (1968) Metabolism of diazepam *in vitro*. Biochem. Pharmacol., 17, 2443-2449

Schwartz, M.A., Koechlin, B.A., Postma, E., Palmer, S. & Krol, G. (1965) Metabolism of diazepam in rat, dog, and man. J. Pharmacol. exp. Ther., 149, 423-435

Schwartz, M.A., Bommer, P. & Vane, F.M. (1967) Diazepam metabolites in the rat: characterization by high-resolution mass spectrometry and nuclear magnetic resonance. Arch. Biochem. Biophys., 121, 508-516

Scott, C.G. & Bommer, P. (1970) The liquid chromatography of some benzo-
    diazepines. J. chromat. Sci., 8, 446-448

Shearer, C.M. & Pilla, C.R. (1974) Oxazepam. In: Florey, K., ed.,
    Analytical Profiles of Drug Substances, Vol. 3, New York, Academic
    Press, pp. 442-464

de Silva, J.A.F. & Puglisi, C.V. (1970) Determination of medazepam
    (nobrium), diazepam (valium) and their major biotransformation
    products in blood and urine by electron capture gas-liquid chromato-
    graphy. Analyt. Chem., 42, 1725-1736

Sisenwine, S.F., Tio, C.O., Shrader, S.R. & Ruelius, H.W. (1972) The bio-
    transformation of oxazepam (7-chloro-1,3-dihydro-3-hydroxy-5-phenyl-
    2H-1,4-benzodiazepin-2-one) in man, miniature swine and rat.
    Arzneimittel-Forsch., 22, 682-687

Stecher, P.G., ed. (1968) The Merck Index, 8th ed., Rahway, NJ, Merck &
    Co., pp. 341, 772-773

Sternbach, L.H. & Reeder, E. (1961) Quinazolines and 1,4-benzodiazepines.
    IV. Transformations of 7-chloro-2-methylamino-5-phenyl-3H-1,4-benzo-
    diazepine 4-oxide. J. org. Chem., 26, 4936-4941

Sternbach, L.H., Reeder, E., Keller, O. & Metlesics, W. (1961) Quinazolines
    and 1,4-benzodiazepines. III. Substituted 2-amino-5-phenyl-3H-1,4-
    benzodiazepine 4 oxides. J. org. Chem., 26, 4488-4497

Steyn, J.M. & Hundt, H.K.L. (1975) Quantitative gas chromatographic deter-
    mination of diazepam and its major metabolite in human serum.
    J. Chromat., 107, 196-200

US Drug Enforcement Administration (1975) Schedules of controlled substances.
    Federal Register, 40, 4016-4017

US Drug Enforcement Administration (1976) Schedules of controlled substances.
    US Code of Federal Regulations, Title 21, 1308.14

US International Trade Commission (1976a) Synthetic Organic Chemicals, US
    Production and Sales, 1974, USITC Publication 776, Washington DC,
    US Government Printing Office, p. 106

US International Trade Commission (1976b) Imports of Benzenoid Chemicals
    and Products, 1974, USITC Publication 762, Washington DC, US Government
    Printing Office, p. 81

US Pharmacopeial Convention, Inc. (1975) The US Pharmacopeia, 19th rev.,
    Rockville, Md, pp. 135-136

US Tariff Commission (1964) Synthetic Organic Chemicals, US Production and
    Sales, 1963, TC Publication 143, Washington DC, US Government Printing
    Office, p. 129

US Tariff Commission (1967) <u>Synthetic Organic Chemicals, US Production and Sales, 1965</u>, TC Publication 206, Washington DC, US Government Printing Office, p. 123

US Tariff Commission (1974) <u>Imports of Benzenoid Chemicals and Products, 1973</u>, TC Publication 688, Washington DC, US Government Printing Office, p. 82

Walkenstein, S.S., Wiser, R., Gudmundsen, C.H., Kimmel, H.B. & Corradino, R.A. (1964) Absorption, metabolism, and excretion of oxazepam and its succinate half-ester. <u>J. pharm. Sci.</u>, <u>53</u>, 1181-1186

Walker, B.E. & Patterson, A. (1974) Induction of cleft palate in mice by tranquilizers and barbiturates. <u>Teratology</u>, <u>10</u>, 159-164

Woodbury, D.M. & Fingl, E. (1975) <u>Drugs effective in the therapy of the epilepsies</u>. In: Goodman, L.S. & Gilman, A., eds, <u>The Pharmacological Basis of Therapeutics</u>, 5th ed., New York, Macmillan, pp. 216-218

DITHRANOL

1. Chemical and Physical Data

1.1 Synonyms and trade names

Chem. Abstr. Reg. Serial No.: 480-22-8

Chem. Abstr. Name: 1,8,9-Anthracenetriol

Anthralin; 1,8,9-anthratriol; 1,8-dihydroxyanthranol; 1,8-dihydroxy-9-anthranol; dioxyanthranol; 1,8,9-trihydroxyanthracene

Anthra-Derm; Batidrol; Chrysodermol; Cignolin; Cigthranol; Cygnolin; Dermaline; Derobin; Lasan; Psoriacid-Stift

1.2 Chemical formula and molecular weight

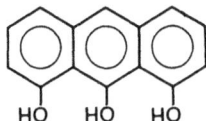

$C_{14}H_{10}O_3$ Mol. wt: 226.2

1.3 Chemical and physical properties of the pure substance

From Stecher (1968), unless otherwise specified

(a) Description: Yellow leaflets or needles

(b) Melting-point: 176-181°C

(c) Spectroscopy data: λ_{max} 256 and 288 nm (E_1^1 = 504 and 411) in methanol; infra-red and nuclear magnetic resonance spectra are also given (Grasselli, 1973)

(d) Solubility: Practically insoluble in water; freely soluble in chloroform; soluble in acetone, benzene, pyridine, oils and dilute sodium hydroxide; slightly soluble in ethanol, ether and glacial acetic acid

(e) Reactivity: When oxidized it produces dithranol dimer and 1,8-dihydroxyanthraquinone in acetone or methanol (Segal *et al.*, 1971)

1.4 Technical products and impurities

Various national and international pharmacopoeias give specifications for the purity of dithranol in pharmaceutical products. For example, dithranol is available in the US as a USP grade containing 95.0-100.5% active ingredient on a dried basis. It is available in ointment form containing 0.1, 0.2, 0.25, 0.4, 0.5 or 1.0% dithranol in a petrolatum or other suitable base which contains 90-115% of the stated amount of dithranol (US Pharmacopeial Convention, Inc., 1975).

In the UK, dithranol is available as an ointment containing 0.1% dithranol in paraffin and containing 90-110% of the stated amount of active ingredient (British Pharmacopoeia Commission, 1973).

2. Production, Use, Occurrence and Analysis

For important background information on this section, see preamble, p. 15.

2.1 Production and use

(a) Production

A method for the synthesis of dithranol by the reduction of 1,8-dihydroxyanthraquinone with hydrogen and nickel catalysts at high pressure was reported in 1938 (Zahn & Koch, 1938). Dithranol can also be prepared by sulphonating anthraquinone and heating the resulting 1,8-disulphonic acid with a calcium hydroxide/calcium chloride mixture to give 1,8-dihydroxyanthraquinone, which is reduced with tin and hydrochloric acid (Harvey, 1975a).

Commercial production of dithranol was first reported in the US in 1936 (US Tariff Commission, 1938). However, since 1957, when it was reported for the last time, dithranol has not been produced in commercial quantities in the US (US Tariff Commission, 1958). US imports through the principal customs districts were 30 kg in 1972 and in 1973 (US Tariff Commission, 1973, 1974) and 120 kg in 1974 (US International Trade Commission, 1976).

(b) Use

Dithranol is a polyphenol with mild skin irritant and antibacterial activity. It is used in human medicine for the treatment of psoriasis and chronic dermatoses (Harvey, 1975b). Dithranol is applied to the skin as an ointment containing from 0.1-1.0% dithranol. The usual dosage regimen begins with the lower available concentration and is increased gradually as needed to obtain the desired therapeutic effect (American Society of Hospital Pharmacists, 1959).

Total US use of dithranol in human medicine is estimated to be less than 25 kg annually.

Dithranol has also been used in veterinary medicine to treat ringworm (Stecher, 1968).

2.2 Occurrence

Dithranol is not known to occur in nature. A chemical closely related to dithranol, 1,8-dihydroxy-3-methyl-9-anthrone, constitutes about 30% of a natural product, chrysarobin (purified Goa powder, purified araroba), which may produce conjunctivitis if used in the treatment of psoriasis (Stecher, 1968).

2.2 Analysis

Methods of assay of dithranol that meet regulatory requirements for pharmaceutical products include UV spectrophotometry and colorimetry. One assay procedure is based on the bromination of dithranol with potassium bromide and potassium bromate (Ionescu-Solomon *et al.*, 1966).

3. Biological Data Relevant to the Evaluation of Carcinogenic Risk to Man

3.1 Carcinogenicity and related studies in animals

Skin administration

Mouse: Groups of 10-16 ICR Swiss or C57/St adult mice, 55 days of age, received a single application of 125 µg 7,12-dimethylbenz[*a*]anthracene (DMBA) in acetone as an initiator; 25 days later they received repeated skin paintings of 0.25 ml of a 0.01% or 0.033% solution of dithranol in acetone 5 times per week for 32 or 48 weeks. In Swiss mice painted 5 times weekly for 48 weeks, the incidences of skin papillomas were 14% (2/14) in animals receiving 0.01%, and 87% (13/15) in animals receiving 0.033% dithranol.

C57/St mice painted with a 0.033% solution developed tumours, with an incidence of 46% (6/13) [P<0.01]. The first tumour appeared 14 weeks after the first application of dithranol. No tumours were observed in C57/St mice painted with a 0.01% solution or in 29 control mice of both strains combined painted with DMBA followed by acetone without the initiator. Applications of dithranol in acetone gave rise to a single skin papilloma among 30 Swiss mice, and no skin tumours occurred among 39 C57/St mice treated with dithranol in acetone. In Swiss mice given one application of dithranol (0.033 or 0.1%) following DMBA initiation, the incidences of skin tumours were 2/15 and 5/15, respectively. Of 36 tumour-bearing mice treated with DMBA and dithranol, 8 developed squamous-cell carcinomas (Bock & Burns, 1963).

A group of 20 7-week old female ICR/Ha mice were painted with a single application of 20 µg DMBA in 0.1 ml acetone, followed 2 weeks later by repeated paintings 3 times weekly for 490 days with 0.1 ml of a 0.08% solution of dithranol in acetone. The first papilloma appeared 59 days after the first application of dithranol. In all, 18 mice developed a total of 94 skin tumours, including 9 squamous-cell carcinomas. In control animals painted with DMBA followed by acetone or by transformation products of dithranol, i.e., dithranol dimer or 1,8-dihydroxyanthraquinone, no tumours were found. Applications of dithranol in acetone without DMBA induced a skin papilloma in 1/20 mice 287 days after the first application of dithranol (Segal *et al.*, 1971).

Groups of 40 and 20 ICR and 20 CFW mice (6 or 8 weeks of age) received i.p. injections of urethane (ethyl carbamate) as initiator in a single dose of 50 mg or as three daily doses of 40 mg, followed 3 days later by repeated skin paintings, 5 times weekly for 27-28 weeks, with 0.25 ml of a 0.033% or 0.1% solution of dithranol in acetone. The cumulative percentages of skin papilloma-bearing mice of both strains pretreated with 3 injections of urethane followed by 0.1% dithranol in acetone were 40% in ICR and 75% in CFW mice. Only one skin tumour was observed in a group of 20 CFW mice treated only with 0.1% dithranol in acetone, and no tumours were observed in a group treated with urethane followed by acetone. Lymphomas were also found in ICR mice: 21/40 mice (52.5%) treated with 50 mg urethane, followed by topical application of 0.033% dithranol in acetone, had developed such tumours when the animals were killed 27 weeks after the start of the experiment; 6/40 (15%) and 4/20 mice (20%) developed lymphomas following topical applications of 0.033% and 0.1% dithranol in acetone without urethane pretreatment; 3/40 (7%) and 4/20 mice (20%) developed lymphomas after treatment with urethane alone at a single dose of 50 mg or three doses of 40 mg (Yasuhira, 1968a,b).

3.2 Other relevant biological data

(a) Experimental systems

Dithranol forms molecular complexes with calf thymus DNA *in vitro* (Swanbeck & Zetterberg, 1971). It induces petite mutants in *Saccharomyces cerevisiae* (Gillberg *et al.*, 1967; Siebert *et al.*, 1970) but no gene conversion in *Saccharomyces cerevisiae* (D4 strain) (Siebert *et al.*, 1970). At the maximum non-toxic dose, no point mutations were found in *Salmonella typhimurium* TA98, TA100, TA1535 or TA1537 in the presence or absence of rat liver homogenate (McCann *et al.*, 1975). In a large mutagenicity study on anthraquinone derivatives, dithranol at near toxic concentrations was negative (or very weak) in inducing point mutations in *Salmonella typhimurium* TA1537, TA98 and TA1538 in the presence of rat liver homogenate (Brown & Brown, 1976).

(b) Man

No changes in liver or kidney function or in the blood picture were observed in 40 patients treated with 0.1-0.4% dithranol paste or ointment topically during the treatment of psoriasis over a 3-month period (Gay *et al.*, 1972). Inhibition of DNA repair after UV irradiation has been reported in cultured peripheral human leucocytes (Gaudin *et al.*, 1972), but this appears to be the result of general cellular toxicity (Cleaver & Painter, 1975; Poirier *et al.*, 1975).

3.3 Case reports and epidemiological studies

No data were available to the Working Group.

4. Comments on Data Reported and Evaluation[1]

4.1 Animal data

Dithranol is a tumour-promoting agent in mouse skin carcinogenesis experiments following initiation with either 7,12-dimethylbenz[*a*]anthracene or urethane. An increased incidence of lymphomas was also observed in mice painted with dithranol after urethane initiation.

4.2 Human data

No case reports or epidemiological studies were available to the Working Group.

---

[1]See also the section 'Animal Data in Relation to the Evaluation of Risk to Man' in the introduction to this volume, p. 13.

5. References

American Society of Hospital Pharmacists (1959) *American Hospital Formulary Service*, Section 84:28, Washington DC

Bock, F.G. & Burns, R. (1963) Tumor-promoting properties of anthralin (1,8,9-anthratriol). *J. nat. Cancer Inst.*, **30**, 393-397

British Pharmacopoeia Commission (1973) *British Pharmacopoeia*, London, HMSO, p. 176

Brown, J.P. & Brown, R.J. (1976) Mutagenesis by 9,10-anthraquinone derivatives and related compounds in *Salmonella typhimurium*. *Mutation Res.*, **40**, 203-224

Cleaver, J.E. & Painter, R.B. (1975) Absence of specificity in inhibition of DNA repair replication by DNA-binding agents, cocarcinogens and steroids in human cells. *Cancer Res.*, **35**, 1773-1778

Gaudin, D., Gregg, R.S. & Yielding, K.L. (1972) Inhibition of DNA repair by cocarcinogens. *Biochem. biophys. Res. Commun.*, **48**, 945-949

Gay, M.W., Moore, W.J., Morgan, J.M. & Montes, L.F. (1972) Anthralin toxicity. *Arch. Dermatol.*, **105**, 213-215

Gillberg, B.O., Zetterberg, G. & Swanbeck, G. (1967) Petite mutants induced in yeast by dithranol (1,8,9-trihydroxyanthracene), an important therapeutic agent against psoriasis. *Nature (Lond.)*, **214**, 415

Grasselli, J.G., ed. (1973) *CRC Atlas of Spectral Data and Physical Constants for Organic Compounds*, Cleveland, Ohio, Chemical Rubber Co., p. B-166

Harvey, S.C. (1975a) Topical drugs. In: Osol, A., *et al.*, eds, *Remington's Pharmaceutical Sciences*, 15th ed., Easton, Pa, Mack, p. 720

Harvey, S.C. (1975b) Antiseptics and disinfectants; fungicides; ectoparasiticides. In: Goodman, L.S. & Gilman, A., eds, *The Pharmacological Basis of Therapeutics*, 5th ed., New York, Macmillan, p. 1006

Ionescu-Solomon, I., Constantinescu, T., Enache, S. & Gamenti, V. (1966) Determination of the product Cignolin - a volumetric method for the determination of 1,8-dihydroxy-9-anthranol. *Rev. Chim. (Buc.)*, **17**, 490-493

McCann, J., Choi, E., Yamasaki, E. & Ames, B.N. (1975) Detection of carcinogens as mutagens in the *Salmonella*/microsome test: assay of 300 chemicals. *Proc. Nat. Acad. Sci. (Wash.)*, **72**, 5135-5139

Poirier, M.C., De Cicco, B.T. & Lieberman, M.W. (1975) Nonspecific inhibition of DNA repair synthesis by tumor promoters in human diploid fibroblasts damaged with N-acetoxy-2-acetylaminofluorene. Cancer Res., 35, 1392-1397

Segal, A., Katz, C. & Van Duuren, B.L. (1971) Structure and tumor-promoting activity of anthralin (1,8-dihydroxy-9-anthrone) and related compounds. J. med. Chem., 14, 1152-1154

Siebert, D., Zimmermann, F.K. & Lemperle, E. (1970) Genetic effects of fungicides. Mutation Res., 10, 533-543

Stecher, P.G., ed. (1968) The Merck Index, 8th ed., Rahway, NJ, Merck & Co., pp. 260, 394

Swanbeck, G. & Zetterberg, G. (1971) Studies on dithranol and dithranol-like compounds. I. Binding to nucleic acids. Acta derm. venereol. (Stockh.), 51, 41-44

US International Trade Commission (1976) Imports of Benzenoid Chemicals and Products, 1974, USITC Publication 762, Washington DC, US Government Printing Office, p. 79

US Pharmacopeial Convention, Inc. (1975) The US Pharmacopeia, 19th rev., Rockville, Md, p. 33

US Tariff Commission (1938) Dyes and Other Synthetic Organic Chemicals in the US, 1936, Report No. 125, Second Series, Washington DC, US Government Printing Office, p. 39

US Tariff Commission (1958) Synthetic Organic Chemicals, US Production and Sales, 1957, Report No. 203, Second Series, Washington DC, US Government Printing Office, p. 103

US Tariff Commission (1973) Imports of Benzenoid Chemicals and Products, 1972, TC Publication 601, Washington DC, US Government Printing Office, p. 82

US Tariff Commission (1974) Imports of Benzenoid Chemicals and Products, 1973, TC Publication 688, Washington DC, US Government Printing Office, p. 78

Yasuhira, K. (1968a) Skin papilloma production by anthralin painting after urethan initiation in mice. Gann, 59, 187-193

Yasuhira, K. (1968b) Induction of malignant lymphoma and other tumors during experiments with anthralin painting of mice. Gann, 59, 195-200

Zahn, K. & Koch, H. (1938) Zur Kenntnis der katalytischen Reduktion und Hydrierung einiger Oxy-anthrachinone. Ber. dtsch. chem. Ges., 71, 172-186

ETHIONAMIDE

1. Chemical and Physical Data

1.1 Synonyms and trade names

Chem. Abstr. Reg. Serial No.: 536-33-4

Chem. Abstr. Name: 2-Ethyl-4-pyridinecarbothioamide

Amidazine; ethina; ethioniamide; α-ethylisonicotinic acid thioamide; 2-ethylisonicotinic acid thioamide; 2-ethylisonicotinic thioamide; α-ethylisonicotinoylthioamide; ethylisothiamide; α-ethylisothionicotinamide; 2-ethylisothionicotinamide; 2-ethyl-4-thioamidylpyridine; 2-ethyl-4-thiocarbamoylpyridine; α-ethylthioisonicotinamide; 2-ethyl-thioisonicotinamide; ethyonamide; thianid; thianide; thioamide

Aetina; Aetiva; Amidazin; Bayer 5312; ETH; Ethinamide; Ethimide; Etimid; Etiocidan; Etionid; Etionizina; Etionizine; ETP; Fatoli-amid; F.I. 58-30; Iridocin; Iridozin; Isothin; Isotiamida; Itiocide; Nicotion; Nisotin; Nizotin; Rigenicid; Sertinon; Teberus; 1314 TH; TH 1314; Th 1314; Thianid; Thioamide; Thiomid; Thioniden; Tio-Mid; Trecator; Trescatyl; Trescazide; Tubermin; Tuberoid; Tuberoson

1.2 Chemical formula and molecular weight

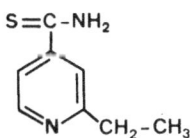

$C_8H_{10}N_2S$ Mol. wt: 166.2

1.3 Chemical and physical properties of the pure substance

From Stecher (1968), unless otherwise specified

(a) Description: Yellow crystals from ethanol

(b) Melting-point: Decomposition at 164-166°C

(c) Spectroscopy data: λ_{max} 290 nm in methanol (US Pharmacopeial Convention, Inc., 1975)

(d) Solubility: Insoluble in water and ether; sparingly soluble in methanol, ethanol and propylene glycol; soluble in hot acetone and ethylene dichloride; freely soluble in pyridine

1.4 Technical products and impurities

Various national and international pharmacopoeias give specifications for the purity of ethionamide in pharmaceutical products. For example, ethionamide is available in the US as a USP grade containing 98.0-102.0% active ingredient on an anhydrous basis, a maximum of 0.003% selenium and 2% water. Tablets are available in a 250 mg dose which contains 95.0-110.0% of the stated amount of ethionamide (US Pharmacopeial Convention, Inc., 1975). In Japan, ethionamide is also available in suppository form. In the UK, it is available in forms containing not less than 98.5% active ingredient on a dried basis and in 125 mg tablets containing 95.0-105.0% of the stated amount of active ingredient (British Pharmacopoeia Commission, 1973).

2. Production, Use, Occurrence and Analysis

For important background information on this section, see preamble, p. 15.

2.1 Production and use

(a) Production

A method of synthesizing ethionamide patented in the UK in 1958 involves dehydration of 2-ethylisonicotinamide to 2-ethylisonicotinonitrile which is reacted with hydrogen sulphide in the presence of triethanolamine to give ethionamide (Chimie et Atomistique, 1958).

Commercial production of ethionamide was first reported in the US in 1968 (US Tariff Commission, 1970); only one US company reported production (see preamble, p. 15) in 1972 (US Tariff Commission, 1974a). US imports of ethionamide through the principal customs districts were about 40 kg in 1972 (US Tariff Commission, 1973), 125 kg in 1973 (US Tariff Commission, 1974b) and 276 kg in 1974 (US International Trade Commission, 1976).

84

(b) Use

Ethionamide is an analogue of thioisonicotinamide and shows strong
antibacterial activity. It is used in human medicine for the treatment of
tuberculosis. It completely suppresses the multiplication of human strains
of *Mycobacterium tuberculosis in vitro* and is usually effective against
bacilli resistant to other tuberculostatic agents. However, since it is
less potent and more toxic than primary antituberculosis drugs, it is used
only as a secondary antituberculosis drug, usually in combination therapy
with primary agents, such as isonicotinic acid hydrazide or streptomycin,
or in cases of primary drug resistance (Weinstein, 1975).

Ethionamide is administered orally at an initial adult dose of
250 mg twice a day. The dosage is increased by 125 mg per day for 5 days
until one gram is administered daily (Weinstein, 1975). The highest tolerated
dose, usually between 750 mg and 1 g per day, is recommended to prevent the
development of resistance (American Society of Hospital Pharmacists, 1963).

2.2 Occurrence

Ethionamide is not known to occur in nature.

2.3 Analysis

Methods of assay of ethionamide that meet regulatory requirements for
pharmaceutical products include titration and UV spectrophotometry.

A simple colorimetric method for its detection and analysis involves
determination of its reaction product with 2,3-dichloro-1,4-naphthoquinone
(Devani *et al.*, 1974). Other colorimetric methods for the determination
of ethionamide in plasma have also been reported (Harnanansingh & Eidus,
1970; Pütter, 1972).

A coulometric assay has been described (Sement *et al.*, 1972).

3. Biological Data Relevant to the Evaluation
of Carcinogenic Risk to Man

3.1 Carcinogenicity and related studies in animals[1]

Oral administration

Mouse: A group of 36 8-week old female BALB/c/Cb/Se mice were given
daily intragastric instillations of 0.1 ml of a 2% solution of ethionamide
in propylene glycol (2 mg/animal) on 6 days per week for 50 weeks; 7/33 mice
surviving 69 weeks developed thyroid tumours (5 papillary and 2 epidermoid
carcinomas) between 28 and 69 weeks. After 69 weeks none of 18 surviving
controls receiving propylene glycol alone and none of 47 untreated controls
had developed thyroid tumours. Five cases of diffuse hypertropy and 3
of nodular hypertrophy were observed in the thyroids of treated mice.
Pulmonary tumours occurred in 7/33 treated mice that died between 60-69
weeks, in 10/38 untreated controls that died between 80-109 weeks and in
2 that died between 40-69 weeks (Biancifiori et al., 1964).

3.2 Other relevant biological data

(a) Experimental systems

The i.p. LD$_{50}$ of ethionamide in mice is 1350 mg/kg bw (Dłuźniewski &
Gastoł-Lewińska, 1971). Intragastric and s.c. administrations of 54 or
270 mg/kg bw ethionamide to pregnant rats on days 6-14 of pregnancy
produced skeletal malformations in their offspring. No malformations were
seen in the offspring of pregnant rabbits treated by gavage with 13.5 or
27.0 mg/kg bw on days 7-14 of pregnancy (Dłuźniewski & Gastoł-Lewińska,
1971).

(b) Man

Toxic hepatitis has been associated with use of ethionamide and is
accompanied by elevated levels of liver enzymes in the plasma (Phillips &
Tashman, 1963; Simon et al., 1969).

---

[1]The Working Group was also aware of on-going studies in mice and
rats (IARC, 1974).

Oral administration of 1 g ethionamide results in peak plasma levels of about 20 μg/ml after 3 hours (Weinstein, 1975). Three metabolic pathways are known: a sulphoxide is formed; the thioketone group is hydrolysed to give 2-ethylpyridine-4-carboxylic acid amide and the free carboxylic acid; or the pyridinium N-atom is methylated, followed by hydroxylation at the 6-carbon atom to give *N*-methyl-2-ethylpyrid-6-one-4-thiocarboxylic acid amide (Bieder & Mazeau, 1962, 1964; Bieder *et al.*, 1966; Iwainsky, 1964; Iwainsky *et al.*, 1965; Kane, 1962; Ritter, 1973). The metabolites were excreted in the urine (Bieder & Brunel, 1971).

3.3 Case reports and epidemiological studies

No data were available to the Working Group.

4. Comments on Data Reported and Evaluation[1]

4.1 Animal data

Ethionamide is carcinogenic in mice after its oral administration, the only species and route of administration tested: it produced thyroid carcinomas.

4.2 Human data

No case reports or epidemiological studies were available to the Working Group.

---

[1]See also the section 'Animal Data in Relation to the Evaluation of Risk to Man' in the introduction to this volume, p. 13.

5. References

American Society of Hospital Pharmacists (1963) American Hospital Formulary Service, section 8:16, Washington DC

Biancifiori, C., Milia, U. & Di Leo, F.P. (1964) Tumori della tiroide indotti mediante etionamide (ET) in topi femmina vergini BALB/c/Cb/Se substrain. Lav. Ist. Anat. Univ. Perugia, 24, 145-166

Bieder, A. & Brunel, P. (1971) Application de la polarographie rapide à courant alternatif surimposé à l'étude de l'élimination urinaire des métabolites de l'éthionamide et du protionamide chez l'homme. Ann. pharm. franç., 29, 461-476

Bieder, A. & Mazeau, L. (1962) Etude du métabolisme de l'éthionamide chez l'homme. I. Séparation des métabolites par chromatographie. Ann. pharm. franç., 20, 211-216

Bieder, A. & Mazeau, L. (1964) Recherches sur le métabolisme de l'éthionamide chez l'homme. Séparation et identification de certains métabolites par chromatographie sur couche mince. Thérapie, 19, 897-907

Bieder, A., Brunel, P. & Mazeau, L. (1966) Identification de trois nouveaux métabolites de l'éthionamide: chromatographie, spectrophotométrie, polarographie. Ann. pharm. franç., 24, 493-500

British Pharmacopoeia Commission (1973) British Pharmacopoeia, London, HMSO, pp. 193-194

Chimie et Atomistique (1958) α-Substituted isonicotinic thioamides. British Patent 800,250, August 20

Devani, M.B., Shishoo, C.J., Mody, H.J. & Raja, P.K. (1974) Detection of thioamides: determination of ethionamide with 2,3-dichloro-1,4-naphthoquinone. J. pharm. Sci., 63, 1471-1473

Dłuźniewski, A. & Gastoł-Lewińska, L. (1971) The search for teratogenic activity of some tuberculostatic drugs. Diss. pharm. (Krakow), 23, 383-392

Harnanansingh, A.M.T. & Eidus, L. (1970) Determination of ethionamide in serum. Int. Z. klin. Pharmakol. Ther. Toxikol., 3, 128-131

IARC (1974) IARC Information Bulletin on the Survey of Chemicals Being Tested for Carcinogenicity, No. 3, Lyon, p. 23

Iwainsky, H. (1964) Zum Stoffwechsel des α-Äthylisonikotinsäurethioamides (Äthioniamid). Z. Tuberkul., 122, 127-130

Iwainsky, H., Sehrt, I. & Grunert, M. (1965) Zum Stoffwechsel des Äthioniamids nach intravenöser Verabreichung. Arzneimittel-forsch., 15, 193-197

Kane, P.O. (1962) Identification of a metabolite of the antituberculous drug ethionamide. Nature (Lond.), 195, 495-496

Phillips, S. & Tashman, H. (1963) Ethionamide jaundice. Amer. Rev. resp. Dis., 87, 896-898

Pütter, J. (1972) Bestimmung von Prothionamid und Äthionamid sowie den entsprechenden Sulfoxiden im Blutplasma. Arzneimittel-Forsch., 22, 1027-1031

Ritter, W. (1973) Neue Ergebnisse über Biotransformation und Pharmako-kinetik von Antituberkulotika. Prax. Pneumol., 27, 139-145

Sement, E., Rousselet, F., Girard, M.L. & Chemla, M. (1972) Les méthodes électrochimiques dans l'analyse pharmaceutique. IV. Applications de la coulométrie à intensité constante au dosage automatique de composés organiques soufrés. Ann. pharm. franç., 30, 691-700

Simon, E., Veres, E. & Bánki, G. (1969) Changes in SGOT activity during treatment with ethionamide. Scand. J. resp. Dis., 50, 314-322

Stecher, P.G., ed. (1968) The Merck Index, 8th ed., Rahway, NJ, Merck & Co., pp. 427-428

US International Trade Commission (1976) Imports of Benzenoid Chemicals and Products, 1974, USITC Publication 762, Washington DC, US Government Printing Office, p. 82

US Pharmacopeial Convention, Inc. (1975) The US Pharmacopeia, 19th rev., Rockville, Md, pp. 187-188

US Tariff Commission (1970) Synthetic Organic Chemicals, US Production and Sales, 1968, TC Publication 327, Washington DC, US Government Printing Office, p. 117

US Tariff Commission (1973) Imports of Benzenoid Chemicals and Products, 1972, TC Publication 601, Washington DC, US Government Printing Office, p. 84

US Tariff Commission (1974a) Synthetic Organic Chemicals, US Production and Sales, 1972, TC Publication 681, Washington DC, US Government Printing Office, p. 110

US Tariff Commission (1974b) Imports of Benzenoid Chemicals and Products, 1973, TC Publication 688, Washington DC, US Government Printing Office, p. 80

Weinstein, L. (1975) Drugs used in the chemotherapy of tuberculosis and leprosy. In: Goodman, L.S. & Gilman, A., eds, The Pharmacological Basis of Therapeutics, 5th ed., New York, Macmillan, pp. 1212-1213

HYCANTHONE and HYCANTHONE MESYLATE

1. Chemical and Physical Data

Hycanthone

1.1 Synonyms and trade names

Chem. Abstr. Reg. Serial No.: 3105-97-3

Chem. Abstr. Name: 1-{[2-(Diethylamino)ethyl]amino}-4-(hydroxy-methyl)-9H-thioxanthen-9-one

1-{[2-(Diethylamino)ethyl]amino}-4-(hydroxymethyl)thioxanthen-9-one; lucanthone metabolite

Win 24933

1.2 Chemical formula and molecular weight

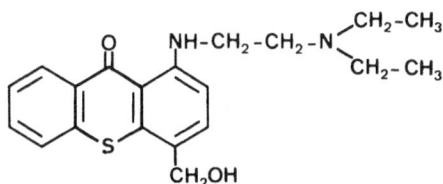

$C_{20}H_{24}N_2O_2S$ Mol. wt: 356.5

1.3 Chemical and physical properties of the pure substance

From Rosi *et al.* (1967) and Blacow (1972)

(a) Description: Orange powder

(b) Melting-point: 100.6-102.8°C

(c) Spectroscopy data: λ_{max} 233, 258, 329 and 428 nm (E_1^1 = 544.2, 1037.9, 272.1 and 185.1) in ethanol

(d) Solubility: Slightly soluble in water

1.4 Technical products and impurities

No information was available to the Working Group.

Hycanthone mesylate

1.1 Synonyms and trade names

Chem. Abstr. Reg. Serial No.: 23255-93-8

Chem. Abstr. Name: 1-{[2-(Diethylamino)ethyl]amino}-4-(hydroxymethyl)-9*H*-thioxanthen-9-one, monomethanesulphonate (salt)

1-{[2-(Diethylamino)ethyl]amino}-4-(hydroxymethyl)thioxanthen-9-one, monomethanesulphonate (salt); hycanthone methanesulphonate; hycanthone monomethanesulphonate

Etrenol

1.2 Chemical formula and molecular weight

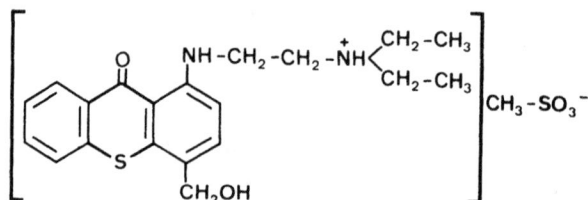

$$C_{21}H_{28}N_2O_5S_2 \qquad \text{Mol. wt: } 452.6$$

1.3 Chemical and physical properties of the pure substance

(a) Description: Yellow-orange powder

(b) Melting-point: About 143°C

(c) Spectroscopy data: λ_{max} 232-234, 257, 327-331 and 428-435 nm in methanol

(d) Solubility: Very soluble in water; freely soluble in 95% ethanol; slightly soluble in chloroform; very slightly soluble in acetone; practically insoluble or insoluble in benzene and ether

(e) Stability: The compound is quite stable; it degrades very rapidly in aqueous-acid solution.

1.4 Technical products and impurities

Hycanthone mesylate is not available commercially in the US but can be obtained in injection form from the Parasitic Disease Drug Service, National Communicable Disease Center, Atlanta, Ga (Swinyard, 1975).

2. Production, Use, Occurrence and Analysis

For important background information on this section, see preamble, p. 15.

2.1 Production and use

(a) Production

Hycanthone is produced by *Aspergillus sclerotiorum* oxidation of the synthetic schistosomicidal drug, lucanthone, and its isolation was first reported in 1965 (Rosi *et al.*, 1965). Hycanthone mesylate was also first produced in 1965 (Rosi *et al.*, 1965); it can be prepared by reacting hycanthone with an equimolar quantity of methanesulphonic acid (Swinyard, 1975).

No evidence was found that hycanthone or hycanthone mesylate have ever been produced commercially in the US or Japan. Both are produced in the UK.

(b) Use

Hycanthone is a schistosomicide effective against human *Schistosoma haemotobium* and *S. mansoni* infections. Given as an intramuscular injection of the mesylate salt, the recommended dose is a single injection of 3.0±0.5 mg hycanthone per kg bw (Friedheim, 1973) to a maximum of 200 mg per injection (Blacow, 1972). Worldwide, over 300,000 patients had been treated with hycanthone mesylate up to June, 1972 (Friedheim, 1973). It is believed that the present number of patients treated is 1.2 million.

2.2 Occurrence

Oxidation of the synthetic drug lucanthone by *Aspergillus sclerotiorum* produces hycanthone, but is not otherwise known to occur in nature (Rosi *et al.*, 1965).

2.3 Analysis

Hycanthone has been determined in urine by thin-layer chromatography (Rosi *et al.*, 1967).

3. Biological Data Relevant to the Evaluation of Carcinogenic Risk to Man

3.1 Carcinogenicity and related studies in animals[1]

Intramuscular administration

Mouse: A group of 66 5-6-week old female CFW mice, infected percuta-neously by tail immersion with 20 *S. mansoni* cercariae, survived for at least 53 weeks; at 54-102 weeks, 19 (29%) had developed diffuse hepatic hyperplasia, 10 (15%) nodular benign hyperplasia and 1 (1.5%) a hepatocellular carcinoma. When a group of 47 mice were similarly infected and treated 56 days later with a single i.m. injection of 3 or 60 mg/kg bw hycanthone mesylate, 33 (70%) developed diffuse hepatic hyperplasia, 12 (26%) nodular benign hyperplasia and 4 (8.5%) hepatocellular carcinomas [P>0.05]. No hepatic hyperplasia or hepatocellular carcinomas developed in any of 45 uninfected mice treated with the same dose of hycanthone or in 47 uninfected, untreated controls (Haese *et al.*, 1973).

Groups of 80-100 4-week old female Swiss Webster mice were infected with either 0, 40 or 80 *S. mansoni* cercariae by i.p. injection; 46 days post-infection the mice were given single i.m. injections of 0, 12.5 or 50 mg/kg bw hycanthone mesylate. While the results proved that hycanthone mesylate was effective in suppressing worms, no evidence was found that the treatment alone or combined with schistosomal infection had any effect on tumour incidence. Only 0-45% of the infected animals survived the 18 months of the experiment (Yarinsky *et al.*, 1974). [The low survival rates in this experiment were noted by the Working Group].

---

[1]The Working Group was aware of ongoing studies in which hycanthone mesylate is being tested in mice and hamsters by i.p. and i.m. injection (IARC, 1976).

Three groups of 144, 59 and 103 female Swiss-Webster CD1 mice were infected by tail immersion with 16 *S. mansoni* cercariae; 8, 12 and 16 weeks after infection they were given three i.m. injections of 0, 3 or 60 mg/kg bw hycanthone. Of 101, 38 and 74 mice in the three groups that survived 60 or more weeks, 0, 1 and 9 (12.2%) developed hepatocellular carcinomas. The increased incidence at the higher dose level was reported to be statistically significant (P=0.001) (Haese & Bueding, 1976).

3.2 Other relevant biological data

(a) Experimental systems

The i.v. LD$_{50}$ of hycanthone in dogs was 40 mg/kg bw; monkeys showed a greater sensitivity than dogs (Henry, 1974). Various adverse biological effects related to hycanthone have been reviewed (de Serres, 1975). It induced hepatoxicity and impaired function of hepatic drug-metabolizing enzymes in rats (Lucier *et al.*, 1973).

In male Sprague-Dawley rats and in rhesus monkeys of both sexes receiving single i.m. injections of randomly tritiated hycanthone mesylate at doses in the range of those therapeutically recommended for man (3 mg/kg bw), peak blood and tissue levels were found about 30-60 minutes after administration. Highest concentrations were observed in the liver, spleen, kidneys and adrenals but decreased to less than 20% of the administered dose in 48-72 hours. Unchanged drug was found in blood and tissues, except in the liver where rapid conversion to hycanthone sulphoxide occurred in rats and to the N-de-ethylated metabolite in monkeys (Hernandez *et al.*, 1971).

In mice, single i.m. doses of 35 or 50 mg/kg bw hycanthone mesylate administered on day 7 of gestation caused malformations in more than 73% of the litters (Moore, 1972). In rabbits, hycanthone mesylate showed embryolethal and teratogenic effects at an i.m. dose of 50 mg/kg bw on days 7, 8 and 9 of gestation (Sieber *et al.*, 1974). The most frequent malformations were exencephaly, hydrocephaly, microphthalmia and abnormalities of the axial skeleton.

The mutagenic properties of hycanthone mesylate have been reviewed (Hartman & Hulbert, 1975). It induces point mutations in *Salmonella typhimurium* TA1538 in the absence of liver homogenate (McCann *et al.*, 1975), sex-linked recessive lethals in *Drosophila melanogaster* (Knaap & Kramers, 1973), mitotic recombination and other mutations in *Saccharomyces cerevisiae* (Meadows *et al.*, 1973; Shahin & de Serres, 1973) and specific locus mutations in the ad-3 region in *Neurospora crassa* (Ong & de Serres, 1975). In mammals, hycanthone has been reported to induce forward mutations at the thymidine kinase locus in mouse lymphoma cells treated with 5-50 μg/ml *in vitro* (Clive *et al.*, 1972). Negative results have been reported in the specific locus test in mice treated with 150 mg/kg bw by i.p. injection (Russell, 1975; Russell & Kelly, 1973) and in the dominant lethal test (cited in Generoso & Cosgrove, 1973; Russell, 1975). Dominant lethals have been reported in rats treated with 40-80 mg/kg bw daily for 5 days by i.p. injection (Green & Springer, 1975; Green *et al.*, 1973a). Cytogenetic effects have also been reported *in vivo* in rat bone-marrow cells (Green *et al.*, 1973b). Hycanthone causes malignant transformation of Rauscher leukaemia virus-infected rat embryo cells but not of non-infected cells (Hetrick & Kos, 1975).

(b) Man

Two of 8 patients treated with a single i.m. injection of 3 mg/kg bw hycanthone for *Schistosoma haematobium* infestation developed severe hepatocellular injury, with the histological pattern of acute toxic hepatitis (Farid *et al.*, 1972).

Cytogenetic effects have been reported in cultures of human peripheral leucocytes treated *in vitro* with hycanthone mesylate (Obe, 1973; Sieber *et al.*, 1973). No chromosome abnormalities were observed in lymphocytes from patients treated with a single injection of 2.5 mg/kg bw hycanthone (Frota-Pessoa *et al.*, 1975).

3.3 Case reports and epidemiological studies

No data were available to the Working Group.

4. Comments on Data Reported and Evaluation[1]

4.1 Animal data

Hycanthone mesylate is carcinogenic in mice previously infected with *Schistosoma mansoni*: a significant increase in the incidence of hepato-cellular carcinomas was observed in these mice following repeated intra-muscular injections of this compound. The limited data available are not sufficient to evaluate whether hycanthone mesylate is carcinogenic in non-infected animals.

4.2 Human data

No case reports or epidemiological studies were available to the Working Group.

---

[1]See also the section 'Animal Data in Relation to the Evaluation of Risk to Man' in the introduction to this volume, p. 13.

5. References

Blacow, N.W., ed. (1972) *Martindale, The Extra Pharmacopoeia*, 26th ed.,
London, Pharmaceutical Press, p. 1617

Clive, D., Flamm, W.G. & Machesko, M.R. (1972) Mutagenicity of hycanthone
in mammalian cells. *Mutation Res.*, *14*, 262-264

Farid, Z., Smith, J.H., Bassily, S. & Sparks, H.A. (1972) Hepatotoxicity
after treatment of schistosomiasis with hycanthone. *Brit. med. J.*,
ii, 88-89

Friedheim, E.A.H. (1973) *Chemotherapy of schistosomiasis.* In: Cavier, R.,
ed., *International Encyclopedia of Pharmacology and Therapeutics*,
Vol. 1, Section 64, *Chemotherapy of Helminthiasis*, New York, Pergamon,
pp. 110-114

Frota-Pessoa, O., Ferreira, N.R., Pedroso, M.B., Moro, A.M., Otto, P.A.,
Chamone, D.A.F. & Da Silva, L.C. (1975) A study of chromosomes of
lymphocytes from patients treated with hycanthone. *J. Toxicol.
environm. Hlth*, *1*, 305-307

Generoso, W.M. & Cosgrove, G.E. (1973) *Total reproductive capacity in female
mice: chemical effects and their analysis.* In: Hollaender, A., ed.,
Chemical Mutagens: Principles and Methods for Their Detection, Vol. 3,
New York, Plenum, pp. 241-258

Green, S. & Springer, J.A. (1975) Additional statistical evaluation and
pharmacological considerations of hycanthone methanesulfonate-induced
dominant lethality. *J. Toxicol. environm. Hlth*, *1*, 293-299

Green, S., Carr, J.V., Sauro, F.M. & Legator, M.S. (1973a) Effects of hycanthone on spermatogonial cells, deoxyribonucleic acid synthesis in bone
marrow and dominant lethality in rats. *J. Pharmacol. exp. Ther.*, *187*,
437-443

Green, S., Sauro, F.M. & Legator, M.S. (1973b) Cytogenetic effects of
hycanthone in the rat. *Mutation Res.*, *17*, 239-244

Haese, W.H. & Bueding, E. (1976) Long-term hepatocellular effects of hycanthone and of two other antischistosomal drugs in mice infected with
Schistosoma mansoni. *J. Pharmacol. exp. Ther.*, *197*, 703-713

Haese, W.H., Smith, D.L. & Bueding, E. (1973) Hycanthone-induced hepatic
changes in mice infected with *Schistosoma mansoni*. *J. Pharmacol. exp.
Ther.*, *186*, 430-440

Hartman, P.E. & Hulbert, P.B. (1975) Genetic activity spectra of some antischistosomal compounds, with particular emphasis on thioxanthenones and
benzothiopyranoindazoles. *J. Toxicol. environm. Hlth*, *1*, 243-270

Henry, M.C. (1974) Preclinical toxicology of hycanthone in dogs and monkeys. NSC 142982, Report 11TR1 TOX 32 PH 43671141, Washington DC, US Government Printing Office

Hernandez, P., Dennis, E.W. & Farah, A. (1971) Metabolism of the schisto-somicidal agent hycanthone by rats and rhesus monkeys. Bull. Wld Hlth Org., 45, 27-34

Hetrick, F.M. & Kos, W.L. (1975) Transformation of cell cultures as a para-meter for detecting the potential carcinogenicity of antischistosomal drugs. J. Toxicol. environm. Hlth, 1, 323-327

IARC (1976) IARC Information Bulletin on the Survey of Chemicals Being Tested for Carcinogenicity, No. 6, Lyon, p. 240

Knaap, A.G.A.C. & Kramers, P.G.N. (1973) Mutagenic effects of hycanthone in Drosophila melanogaster. Mutation Res., 21, 38-39

Lucier, G.W., McDaniel, O.S., Bend, J.R. & Faeder, E. (1973) Effects of hycanthone and two of its chlorinated analogs on hepatic microsomes. J. Pharmacol. exp. Ther., 186, 416-424

McCann, J., Choi, E., Yamasaki, E. & Ames, B.N. (1975) Detection of carcino-gens as mutagens in the Salmonella/microsome test: assay of 300 chemicals. Proc. nat. Acad. Sci. (Wash.), 72, 5135-5139

Meadows, M.G., Quah, S-K. & von Borstel, R.C. (1973) Mutagenic action of hycanthone and IA-4 on yeast. J. Pharmacol. exp. Ther., 187, 444-450

Moore, J.A. (1972) Teratogenicity of hycanthone in mice. Nature (Lond.), 239, 107-109

Obe, G. (1973) Action of hycanthone on human chromosomes in leukocyte cultures. Mutation Res., 21, 287-288

Ong, T-M. & de Serres, F.J. (1975) Mutagenic evaluation of antischistosomal drugs and their derivatives in Neurospora crassa. J. Toxicol. environm. Hlth, 1, 271-279

Rosi, D., Peruzzotti, G., Dennis, E.W., Berberian, D.A., Freele, H. & Archer, S. (1965) A new, active metabolite of 'miracil D'. Nature (Lond.), 208, 1005-1006

Rosi, D., Peruzzotti, G., Dennis, E.W., Berberian, D.A., Freele, H., Tullar, B.F. & Archer, S. (1967) Hycanthone, a new active metabolite of lucanthone. J. med. Chem., 10, 867-876

Russell, W.L. (1975) Results of tests for possible transmitted genetic effects of hycanthone in mammals. J. Toxicol. environm. Hlth, 1, 301-304

Russell, W.L. & Kelly, E.M. (1973) Ineffectiveness of hycanthone in inducing specific-locus mutations in mice. <u>Mutation Res.</u>, <u>21</u>, 14

de Serres, F.J., ed. (1975) Long-term toxicity of antischistosomal drugs. J. Toxicol. environm. Hlth, <u>1</u>

Shahin, M.M. & de Serres, F.J. (1973) The effect of pH on hycanthone methanesulfonate-induced inactivation and mitotic recombination in D5, a new diploid strain of *Saccharomyces cerevisiae*. <u>Mutation Res.</u>, <u>21</u>, 234

Sieber, S.M., Whang-Peng, J., Johns, D.G. & Adamson, R.H. (1973) Effects of hycanthone on rapidly proliferating cells. <u>Biochem. Pharmacol.</u>, <u>22</u>, 1253-1262

Sieber, S.M., Whang-Peng, J. & Adamson, R.H. (1974) Teratogenic and cyto-genetic effects of hycanthone in mice and rabbits. <u>Teratology</u>, <u>10</u>, 227-236

Swinyard, E.A. (1975) <u>Parasiticides</u>. In: Osol, A. *et al.*, eds, <u>Remington's Pharmaceutical Sciences</u>, 15th ed., Easton, Pa, Mack, pp. 1174-1175

Yarinsky, A., Drobeck, H.P., Freele, H., Wiland, J. & Gumaer, K.I. (1974) An 18-month study of the parasitologic and tumorigenic effects of hycanthone in *Schistosoma mansoni*-infected and noninfected mice. <u>Toxicol. appl. Pharmacol.</u>, <u>27</u>, 169-182

8-HYDROXYQUINOLINE

1. Chemical and Physical Data

1.1 Synonyms and trade names

Chem. Abstr. Reg. Serial No.: 148-24-3

Chem. Abstr. Name: 8-Quinolinol

Hydroxybenzopyridine; 8-hydroxy quinoline; oxin; oxine; oxybenzo-pyridine; oxychinolin; 8-oxyquinoline; phenopyridine; 8-quinol

8-OQ; Bioquin; Quinophenol; Tumex

1.2 Chemical formula and molecular weight

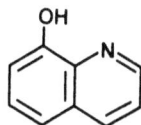

C_9H_7NO Mol. wt: 145.2

1.3 Chemical and physical properties of the pure substance

From Stecher (1968), unless otherwise specified

(a) Description: White crystals or crystalline powder

(b) Boiling-point: About $267^{O}C$

(c) Melting-point: $76^{O}C$

(d) Spectroscopy data: λ_{max} 318 and 243 nm in cyclohexane; infra-red and nuclear magnetic resonance spectra are also given (Grasselli, 1973).

(e) Solubility: Almost insoluble in water and ether; freely soluble in acetone, aqueous mineral acids, benzene, chloroform and ethanol

(f) Reactivity: Readily forms stable metal chelates

1.4 Technical products and impurities

8-Hydroxyquinoline is available in the US in technical and reagent grades. It is also available as a 0.5% solution (or aerosol) suitable for topical use (Harvey, 1975).

2. Production, Use, Occurrence and Analysis

For important background information on this section, see preamble, p. 15.

2.1 Production and use

(a) Production

8-Hydroxyquinoline was first prepared by the decarboxylation of 8-hydroxyquinoline-4-carboxylic acid (Prager & Jacobson, 1935). It has also been prepared by heating 2-aminophenol, glycerine and 2-nitrophenol in concentrated sulphuric acid (Prager & Jacobson, 1935) and by the fusion of quinoline-8-sulphonic acid with caustic soda and water (Bedall & Fischer, 1881). 8-Hydroxyquinoline can also be prepared by the sulphonation of quinoline with oleum and fusion of the sodium salt with sodium hydroxide at $225^{o}C$ (Kulka, 1968).

In the US, commercial production of 8-hydroxyquinoline was first reported in 1933 (US Tariff Commission, 1934); only two US companies reported production (see preamble, p. 15) in 1974 (US International Trade Commission, 1976a). Production of the sulphate salt was reported to be 4,000 kg in 1974 (US International Trade Commission, 1976a). US imports of 8-hydroxyquinoline through the principal customs districts were 25,000 kg in 1972 (US Tariff Commission, 1973), 8000 kg in 1973 (US Tariff Commission, 1974) and 47,000 kg in 1974 (US International Trade Commission, 1976b).

One company produces 8-hydroxyquinoline in Japan, and its annual production is estimated to be in the range of 100-500 thousand kg. Annual production of 8-hydroxyquinoline in western Europe is estimated to be in the range of 0.5-1 million kg, of which 1-100 thousand kg are produced in the Federal Republic of Germany and 100-500 thousand kg in France and in the UK.

(b) Use

8-Hydroxyquinoline is an antimicrobial drug used in human medicine for the treatment of minor burns and haemorrhoids (Harvey, 1975) and has reportedly been used as a bacteriostatic additive in hairdressing preparations to control dandruff (Markland, 1966). Total US sales of the compound for use in human medicine as an antiseptic spray are estimated to be less than 400 kg annually.

As 8-hydroxyquinoline forms a chelate with many metal ions, it is used as an analytical colorimetric reagent and for the precipitation and separation of metals (Stecher, 1968).

8-Hydroxyquinoline is also used in the preparation of a number of derivatives used in medicine and in a variety of industrial applications. The benzoate salt is used in the treatment of minor burns and haemorrhoids and was reportedly a component of a commercial spermicidal preparation (Hoch-Ligeti, 1957). The sulphate salt is used in the treatment of dermatophytosis, vaginitis and as an eyewash and gargle (Harvey, 1975).

8-Hydroxyqinoline is a chemical intermediate for preparation of the amoebacide, diiodohydroxyquin, which may be used in the treatment of intestinal amoebiasis, *Trichomonas vaginalis* vaginitis, infections caused by *Trichomonas hominis*, and in the topical treatment of certain fungal cutaneous infections. Iodochlorhydroxyquin, another derivative of 8-hydroxyquinoline, is used as an antibacterial and antifungal agent in dermatologic preparations and for the treatment of intestinal amoebiasis (Harvey, 1975).

8-Hydroxyquinoline is also used to make its copper chelate, copper 8-hydroxyquinolate, which is registered in the US by the Environmental Protection Agency for use as a fungicide in agricultural and industrial applications.

8-Hydroxyquinoline can also be used in the manufacture of the following dyes: CI Acid Orange 61, CI Mordant Orange 26, CI Direct Black 104, and CI Direct Red 174 (The Society of Dyers and Colourists, 1971); however, no evidence was found that these dyes are produced commercially in the US.

2.2 Occurrence

8-Hydroxyquinoline is not known to occur in nature.

2.3 Analysis

Of 6 colorimetric methods for the determination of 8-hydroxyquinoline in pharmaceutical products and tissues, one using Gibs reagent (2,6-dibromo-benzoquinone chlorimine) was reported to be the most sensitive, with a detection limit of 0.5 µg/l (Galea & Popa, 1971). A colorimetric method for its determination in galenical preparations containing other phenols is based on its complex with a vanadium ion (Peteri, 1969).

Non-aqueous titration methods have been described to determine 8-hydroxyquinoline and its oxidation products (Kondratov *et al.*, 1967) and to determine 8-hydroxyquinoline and some of its metal chelates (Grey & Cave, 1969). An aqueous titration method for the determination of 8-hydroxyquinoline sulphate has been outlined (Horwitz, 1970), and it can be determined fluorimetrically as its chelate compound with tin (2+) (Khabarov *et al.*, 1971). A fluorimetric determination of 8-hydroxyquinoline is based on its luminescence in sulphuric acid at 77^OK and has a sensitivity of 0.12 µM (Golovina *et al.*, 1974).

A spectrophotometric method for the determination of 8-hydroxyquinoline as the copper chelate can be used in the presence of some other metals (Winde, 1970).

Paper, thin-layer and gas-liquid chromatography can also be used to determine 8-hydroxyquinoline (Clarke, 1969).

3. Biological Data Relevant to the Evaluation of Carcinogenic Risk to Man

3.1 Carcinogenicity and related studies in animals

(a) Oral administration

Mouse: A group of 49 CC57W mice were given 1.5 mg/animal 8-hydroxyquinoline in sunflower oil 6 times per week for 660 days (total dose, 852 mg/animal). Of 21 mice surviving at the time of appearance of the first tumour (460 days), 4 developed 2 lymphomas, 2 lung adenomas and 1 haemangioma of the liver. The tumour incidence in untreated CC57W mice in that laboratory was reported to be 17% (Pliss & Volfson, 1970) [The absence of concurrent controls was noted].

Rat: A group of 15 6-week old male Fischer F344 rats received 0.8% 8-hydroxyquinoline in the diet for 78 weeks, at which time 13 survived. The only tumours observed were 4 Leydig-cell tumours of the testis. Hyperplasia of the interstitial cells of the testis was observed in 2/8 surviving controls (Yamamoto et al., 1971) [The small number of animals and the short duration of the experiment were noted].

Groups of male and female Fischer rats were treated with 8-hydroxyquinoline at the following dose levels: 12 males at 0.1 mg/animal/day, 12 females at 3 mg/animal/day, 15 males and 14 females at 10 mg/animal/day and 2 males and 3 females at 30 mg/animal/day. Maximum survival ranged from 384-563 days. One hepatoma with lung metastases occurred after 456 days in one male rat given the highest dose level. No liver tumours occurred in a large number of vehicle or untreated controls. Three cystic adenomas of the lung, 15 testicular tumours and 4 mammary tumours occurred among rats in the other groups; these tumours also occurred in controls surviving up to 600 days. The incidence in treated animals was slightly but not significantly increased (Hadidian et al., 1968).

A group of 39 random-bred rats were given 15 mg/animal 8-hydroxyquinoline in sunflower oil 6 times per week for 729 days (total dose, 9.36 g/animal). Of 21 rats surviving at the time of appearance of the first tumour (589 days), 11 developed 2 lymphomas, 1 lung tumour (plasmocytoma), 2 parasitic sarcomas of the liver, 1 reticulosarcoma of the intestine, 1 adenocarcinoma of the uterus and 5 mammary fibroadenomas. In untreated rats of that laboratory, no tumours of the uterus, lung or intestine or lymphomas were observed (Pliss & Volfson, 1970) [The absence of concurrent controls was noted].

(b) Subcutaneous administration

Mouse: A group of 32 CC57W mice received s.c. injections of 1.5 mg/animal 8-hydroxyquinoline in sunflower oil 3 times per month for 660 days (total dose, 97.5 mg/animal). Of 23 mice surviving at the time of appearance of the first tumour (148 days), 10 developed a total of 2 lymphomas,

5 lung adenomas, 1 subcutaneous haemangioma, 1 follicular adenoma of the ovary and 2 haemangiomas of the liver. In untreated CC57W mice of that laboratory the tumour incidence was reported to be less than 17% (Pliss & Volfson, 1970) [The absence of concurrent controls was noted].

Rat: A group of 70 random-bred rats received weekly s.c. injections of 100 mg/animal 8-hydroxyquinoline in sunflower oil for 730 days (total dose, 10.5 g/animal). Of 24 rats surviving at the appearance of the first tumour (624 days), 4 developed 3 lymphomas and 1 fibrosarcoma at the injection site (Pliss & Volfson, 1970) [The absence of concurrent controls was noted].

(c) Skin application

Mouse: A group of 46 CC57W mice received 3 applications per week of 1.2 mg 8-hydroxyquinoline as a 0.75% solution in benzene for 656 days (total dose, 335 mg/animal). A control group of 22 mice received benzene alone for 656 days. Of 27 treated mice surviving at the appearance of the first tumour (350 days), 8 developed 2 lymphomas, 2 subcutaneous haemangiomas, 1 subcu-taneous lymphangioma, 1 follicular adenoma of the ovary and 2 haemangiomas of the liver; 2/22 control mice receiving benzene alone developed lung adenomas after 427 and 619 days (Pliss & Volfson, 1970) [P>0.05].

(d) Other experimental systems

Bladder implantation: A group of 20 stock mice (sex unspecified) received a bladder implant of a 9-11 mg cholesterol pellet containing 20% 8-hydroxyquinoline. Of 13 mice surviving 40 or more weeks, 5 developed bladder tumours (3 carcinomas and 2 papillomas), compared with 1 carcinoma in 21 controls alive at 40 weeks (P<0.01) (Allen et al., 1957; Boyland & Watson, 1956). Similar results were obtained by Clayson et al. (1958) who observed 6 carcinomas in 25 treated mice compared with 5 in 55 controls. In a further study in which paraffin-wax pellets containing 20% 8-hydroxy-quinoline were implanted into the bladders of 8-13-week old female Swiss mice, 1 papilloma and 1 carcinoma of the bladder were found among 35 treated mice (average survival, 410 days), compared with 1 papilloma and 1 carcinoma among 47 controls given implants of paraffin wax alone (average survival, 366 days) (Bryan et al., 1964).

Vaginal instillation: A group of 20 female stock mice received vaginal instillations of 0.1 ml of a 1% solution of 8-hydroxyquinoline in polyethylene glycol twice weekly for 18 months. Ten mice survived 12 months and 2 for 18 months; 7 developed carcinomas of the vagina and cervix. In controls given polyethylene glycol alone, 11 mice survived for 12 months and 7 for 18 months; 5 developed carcinomas of the vagina and cervix (Boyland et al., 1961). In a later test, 20 BALB/c mice received similar twice weekly instillations of 0.1 ml of a 1% solution of 8-hydroxyquinoline in gum tragacanth for 50 weeks. One mouse developed a squamous papilloma of the uterine cervix after 20 months. No increase in the incidence of tumours at other sites was observed (Boyland et al., 1966).

A group of 46 CC57W mice received twice weekly intravaginal applications of 2 mg/animal 8-hydroxyquinoline as a 20% suspension in distilled water applied to a small piece of cotton wool; treatment continued to 812 days (total dose, 428 mg/animal); 27 controls received an insertion of cotton wool and distilled water. Of 42 treated mice still alive at the time of the appearance of the first tumour (242 days), 11 developed 4 lymphomas, 4 lung adenomas, 5 follicular adenomas and thecomas of the ovary and 1 haemangioma of the liver; 2 lymphomas, 1 lung adenoma and 1 haemangioma of the liver occurred in 27 controls (Pliss & Volfson, 1970) [P>0.05].

A group of 30 female Bethesda black rats received vaginal instillations of 0.2 ml of a 20% suspension of 8-hydroxyquinoline in 20% aqueous gelatin twice weekly for 2 years; 16 rats survived 22-24 months. Four squamous-cell carcinomas or adenocarcinomas of the endometrium were observed in 22 rats that died after 19 months; 1 uterine carcinoma was seen in a group of 21 controls that died between 19 and 24 months (Hueper, 1965) [P>0.05].

A group of 62 random-bred rats received twice weekly intravaginal instillations of 20 mg/animal 8-hydroxyquinoline as a 20% suspension in distilled water; treatment continued for 729 days (total dose, 3.86 g/animal). Of 24 rats still alive at the appearance of the first tumour (647 days), 4 developed 1 lymphoma, 1 follicular adenoma of the ovary, 1 carcinoma of the uterus, 2 mammary fibroadenomas and 1 thyroid carcinoma. In untreated rats of that laboratory, no tumours of the uterus or lymphomas were reported to occur (Pliss & Volfson, 1970) [The absence of concurrent controls was noted].

3.2 Other relevant biological data

(a) Experimental systems

In mice, s.c., oral and painting LD_{50}'s of 8-hydroxyquinoline are 7.5 mg, 7.5 mg and 6 mg/animal, respectively. In rats, s.c. and oral LD_{50}'s are 500 and 75 mg/animal, respectively (Pliss & Volfson, 1970). The oral LD_{20} in guinea-pigs is 1.2 g/kg bw (Stecher, 1968).

In rats, orally administered 8-hydroxyquinoline produced a deposition of iron in many tissues (Yamamoto *et al.*, 1971); this effect was increased by increasing the amount of available iron in the diet (Williams & Yamamoto, 1972).

8-Hydroxyquinoline, at a dose of 20-40 µg/plate, caused point mutations in *Salmonella typhimurium* TA100 in the presence of rat liver homogenate (Talcott *et al.*, 1976). In a brief note, in which control values were not reported, a variety of chromosome abnormalities were reported in mouse bone-marrow cells after treatment with 40 mg/kg bw by i.p. injection (Das & Manna, 1970).

(b) Man

No data were available to the Working Group.

3.3 Case reports and epidemiological studies

No data were available to the Working Group.

4. Comments on Data Reported and Evaluation[1]

4.1 Animal data

8-Hydroxyquinoline has been tested in mice and rats by oral, subcutaneous and intravaginal administration and in mice by skin application and bladder implantation. Most of these experiments were of limited value, for the reasons mentioned in the text. Within these limitations, the

---

[1]Data on the copper chelate of 8-hydroxyquinoline were discussed, but because its chemical properties and uses are different from those of 8-hydroxyquinoline it will be considered by a further Working Group.

studies in mice and rats by oral administration and subcutaneous injection or in mice by skin application gave positive or negative results of borderline significance.

Positive results were obtained in bladder implantation experiments when 8-hydroxyquinoline was incorporated in cholesterol pellets but were negative when paraffin wax pellets were employed (see also introduction, p. 19). **Its application intravaginally in different vehicles to mice and** rats did not significantly increase the incidence of tumours when compared with that in appropriate controls.

No evaluation of the carcinogenicity of 8-hydroxyquinoline can be made on the basis of the available data (however, see also the results obtained in mutagenicity studies).

4.2 Human data

No case reports or epidemiological studies were available to the Working Group.

5. References

Allen, M.J., Boyland, E., Dukes, C.E., Horning, E.S. & Watson, J.G. (1957) Cancer of the urinary bladder induced in mice with metabolites of aromatic amines and tryptophan. Brit. J. Cancer, 11, 212-228

Bedall, K. & Fischer, O. (1881) Über Oxychinolin aus Chinolinsulfosäure. Ber. dtsch. chem. Ges., 14, 442-443, 1366-1369

Boyland, E. & Watson, G. (1956) 3-Hydroxyanthranilic acid, a carcinogen produced by endogenous metabolism. Nature (Lond.), 177, 837-838

Boyland, E., Charles, R.T. & Gowing, N.F.C. (1961) The induction of tumours in mice by intravaginal application of chemical compounds. Brit. J. Cancer, 15, 252-256

Boyland, E., Roe, F.J.C. & Mitchley, B.C.V. (1966) Test of certain constituents of spermicides for carcinogenicity in genital tract of female mice. Brit. J. Cancer, 20, 184-189

Bryan, G.T., Brown, R.R. & Price, J.M. (1964) Incidence of mouse bladder tumors following implantation of paraffin pellets containing certain tryptophan metabolites. Cancer Res., 24, 582-585

Clarke, E.G.C., ed. (1969) Isolation and Identification of Drugs in Pharmaceuticals, Body Fluids and Post-mortem Material, London, Pharmaceutical Press, pp. 375-376

Clayson, D.B., Jull, J.W. & Bonser, G.M. (1958) The testing of *ortho* hydroxyamines and related compounds by bladder implantation and a discussion of their structural requirements for carcinogenic activity. Brit. J. Cancer, 12, 222-230

Das, R.K. & Manna, G.K. (1970) Chromosome aberrations in the bone marrow cells of mice induced by 8-hydroxyquinoline. In: Proceedings of the 57th Indian Science Congress, part III, Section VII, Zoology and Entomology, p. 354

Galea, V. & Popa, L. (1971) Analysis of oxine and its derivatives. Farmacia (Buc.), 19, 17-23

Golovina, A.P., Runov, V.K. & Alimarin, I.P. (1974) Luminescence of 8-hydroxyquinoline. Izv. Akad. Nauk SSSR, Ser. Khim., 6, 1425-1427

Grasselli, J.G., ed. (1973) CRC Atlas of Spectral Data and Physical Constants for Organic Compounds, Cleveland, Ohio, Chemical Rubber Co., p. B-876

Grey, P. & Cave, G.C.B. (1969) Chelate-exchange titrimetry in non-aqueous solvents. II. Determination of 8-quinolinol and metal 8-quinolinates. Canad. J. Chem., 47, 4555-4562

Hadidian, Z., Fredrickson, T.N., Weisburger, E.K., Weisburger, J.H., Glass, R.M. & Mantel, N. (1968)   Tests for chemical carcinogens. Report on the activity of derivatives of aromatic amines, nitrosamines, quinolines, nitroalkanes, amides, epoxides, aziridines and pure anti-metabolites.   J. nat. Cancer Inst., 41, 985-1036

Harvey, S.C. (1975)   Antimicrobial drugs.   In: Osol, A. et al., eds, Remington's Pharmaceutical Sciences, 15th ed., Easton, Pa, Mack, pp. 1093, 1103, 1159

Hoch-Ligeti, C. (1957)   Effect of prolonged administration of spermicidal contraceptives on rats kept on low-protein or on full diet.   J. nat. Cancer Inst., 18, 661-685

Horwitz, W., ed. (1970)   Official Methods of Analysis of the Association of Official Analytical Chemists, 11th ed., Washington DC, Association of Official Analytical Chemists, p. 697

Hueper, W.C. (1965)   Experimental studies on 8-hydroxyquinoline in rats and mice.   Arch. Pathol., 79, 245-250

Khabarov, A.A., Shemyakin, F.M. & Fakeeva, O.A. (1971)   Fluorometric determination of 8-hydroxyquinoline, 4- and 8-aminoquinoline, and cinchoninic acid derivatives.   Novye Metody Khim. Anal. Mater., 2, 95-97

Kondratov, V.K., Rus'yanova, N.D., Malysheva, N.V. & Yurkina, L.P. (1967)   Determination of pyridine and quinoline basis in mixtures with their oxidation products.   Zh. analyt. Khim., 22, 1585-1589

Kulka, M. (1968)   Quinoline and isoquinoline.   In: Kirk, R.E. & Othmer, D.F., eds, Encyclopedia of Chemical Technology, 2nd ed., Vol. 16, New York, John Wiley and Sons, pp. 865-886

Markland, W.R. (1966)   Hair preparations.   In: Kirk, R.E. & Othmer, D.F., eds, Encyclopedia of Chemical Technology, 2nd ed., Vol. 10, New York, John Wiley and Sons, p. 780

Peteri, D. (1969)   Photometric determination of 8-hydroxyquinoline in the presence of other phenols in galenical preparations.   Fresenius' Z. analyt. Chem., 248, 38-39

Pliss, G.B. & Volfson, N.I. (1970)   On carcinogenic action of 8-hydroxyquinoline.   Vop. Onkol., 16, 67-71

Prager, B. & Jacobson, P., eds (1935)   Beilsteins Handbuch der organischen Chemie, 4th ed., Vol. 21, Syst. No. 3114, Berlin, Springer-Verlag, p. 91

The Society of Dyers and Colourists (1971)   Colour Index, 3rd ed., Vol. 4, Bradford, Yorks, pp. 4134, 4264

Stecher, P.G., ed. (1968) The Merck Index, 8th ed., Rahway, NJ, Merck & Co., p. 555

Talcott, R., Hollstein, M. & Wei, E. (1976) Mutagenicity of 8-hydroxyquinoline and related compounds in the *Salmonella typhimurium* bioassay. Biochem. Pharmacol., 25, 1323-1328

US International Trade Commission (1976a) Synthetic Organic Chemicals, US Production and Sales, 1974, USITC Publication 776, Washington DC, US Government Printing Office, pp. 95, 101, 103

US International Trade Commission (1976b) Imports of Benzenoid Chemicals and Products, 1974, USITC Publication 762, Washington DC, US Government Printing Office, p. 26

US Tariff Commission (1934) Production and Sales of Dyes and Other Synthetic Organic Chemicals, 1933, Report No. 89, Second Series, Washington DC, US Government Printing Office, p. 32

US Tariff Commission (1973) Imports of Benzenoid Chemicals and Products, 1972, TC Publication 601, Washington DC, US Government Printing Office, p. 22

US Tariff Commission (1974) Imports of Benzenoid Chemicals and Products, 1973, TC Publication 688, Washington DC, US Government Printing Office, p. 22

Williams, G.M. & Yamamoto, R.S. (1972) Absence of stainable iron from preneoplastic and neoplastic lesions in rat liver with 8-hydroxyquinolineinduced siderosis. J. nat. Cancer Inst., 49, 685-692

Winde, E. (1970) Quantitative determination of 8-hydroxyquinoline. Dtsch. Apoth.-Ztg., 110, 123-124

Yamamoto, R.S., Williams, G.M., Frankel, H.H. & Weisburger, J.H. (1971) 8-Hydroxyquinoline: chronic toxicity and inhibitory effect on the carcinogenicity of *N*-2-fluorenylacetamide. Toxicol. appl. Pharmacol., 19, 687-698

1. Chemical and Physical Data

1.1 Synonyms and trade names

Chem. Abstr. Reg. Serial No.: 443-48-1

Chem. Abstr. Name: 2-Methyl-5-nitro-1H-imidazole-1-ethanol

1-(β-Ethylol)-2-methyl-5-nitro-3-azapyrrole; 1-hydroxyethyl-2-methyl-5-nitroimidazole; 1-(2-hydroxyethyl)-2-methyl-5-nitroimidazole; 1-(β-hydroxyethyl)-2-methyl-5-nitroimidazole; 2-methyl-5-nitro-1-imidazoleethanol; 2-methyl-5-nitroimidazole-1-ethanol

Acromona; Anagiardil; Atrivyl; Bayer 5360; Bexon; Clont; Cont; Danizol; Deflamon-Wirkstoff; Efloran; Elyzol; Entizol; Eumin; Flagemona; Flagesol; Flagil; Flagyl; Flegyl; Giatricol; Gineflavir; Klion; Maxibol 'silanes'; Meronidal; Metronidaz; Metronidazol; Monagyl; Nalox; Neo-Tric; Nida; Novonidazol; Orvagil; RP 8823; Sanatrichom; SC 10295; Takimetol; Trichazol; Trichex; Trichocide; Trichomol; Trichomonacid 'Pharmachim'; Trichopal; Trichopol; Tricocet; Tricom; Tricowas B; Trikacide; Trikamon; Trikojol; Trikozol; Trimeks; Trivazol; Vagilen; Vagimid; Vertisal

1.2 Chemical formula and molecular weight

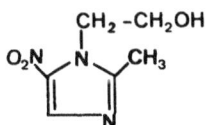

$C_6H_9N_3O_3$ Mol. wt: 171.2

1.3 Chemical and physical properties of the pure substance

From Stecher (1968), unless other specified

(a) Description: Cream crystals

(b) Melting-point: 160°C

(c) Spectroscopy data: Infra-red spectrum is given by Stambaugh et $al.$ (1968)

(d) Solubility: Soluble at 20°C in water (1 g/100 ml), in ethanol
     (0.5 g/100 ml), in ether (<0.05 g/100 ml) and in chloroform
     (<0.05 g/100 ml); sparingly soluble in dimethylformamide;
     soluble in dilute acids

1.4 Technical products and impurities

Various national and international pharmacopoeias give specifications
for the purity of metronidazole in pharmaceutical products. For example,
metronidazole is available in the US as a USP grade containing 99-101%
active ingredient on a dried basis and not more than 0.005% heavy metals.
Suppositories in 500 mg doses and tablets in 250 mg doses contain 95-105%
of the stated amount of metronidazole (US Pharmacopeial Convention, Inc.,
1975).

It is available in the UK on a dried basis containing 99-101% active
ingredient and as 200 mg tablets containing 95-105% of the stated amount
(British Pharmacopoeia Commission, 1973).

2. Production, Use, Occurrence and Analysis

For important background information on this section, see preamble,
p. 15.

2.1 Production and use

(a) Production

A method for the synthesis of metronidazole was patented in the US in
1960 in which 2-methyl-4(or 5)-nitroimidazole is heated with ethylene
chlorohydrin, and the isolated crude metronidazole is recrystallized from
ethyl acetate (Jacob *et al.*, 1960).

Commercial production of metronidazole was first reported in the US in
1963 (US Tariff Commission, 1964); only one US company reported production
(see preamble, p. 15) in 1974 (US International Trade Commission, 1976).

Japanese production of metronidazole was first reported in 1961. In
1975, one Japanese company reported production of 2100 kg, and imports
from France and Canada were reported to be 385 kg. Annual production is
estimated to be 1-100 thousand kg in both Italy and the UK.

India was reported to have one producer of metronidazole in 1972, with a production volume of 6,922 kg. Indian imports for the period 1972-1973 were reported to be 16,250 kg (Anon., 1974).

(b) Use

Metronidazole is effective on oral administration in infections due to *Entamoeba histolytica*, *Trichomonas vaginalis* and *Giardia lamblia* and has been used in Vincent's infection (Blacow, 1972). It is prescribed for invasive intestinal amoebiasis or amoebic hepatic abscess. One recommended oral dose regime is 750 mg three times per day for 5 to 10 days (Rollo, 1975a).

Metronidazole was shown to be an effective systemic trichomonacidal agent in 1960. It imparts trichomonacidal activity to semen and urine, and a high cure rate can be obtained in both male and female patients infected with *Trichomonas vaginalis*. A currently accepted dose regime is 250 mg metronidazole orally three times per day for 7 days. Stubborn infections can be treated by a repeated course, but an interval of 4 to 6 weeks is recommended between treatments (Rollo, 1975b; US Food & Drug Administration, 1976). It can also be applied in pessaries, in a dose of 500 mg daily for 10-20 days (Blacow, 1972).

In giardiasis, a daily dose of 500 mg for 5 days, repeated if necessary, is usually effective (Blacow, 1972).

Metronidazole has been evaluated for use in the treatment of alcoholism (Blacow, 1972), and in the USSR, indications for such use are given (Mashkovski, 1972).

The use of metronidazole in the treatment of acne rosacea has been suggested recently (Pye & Burton, 1976), and a good clinical response was also reported to occur in a small number of patients with acne vulgaris (Carne, 1976).

In early 1976, the US Food and Drug Administration announced that, in future, all packages of metronidazole offered for sale in the US would be required to carry a warning label stating that unnecessary use of the drug should be avoided in view of the results of animal carcinogenicity studies (see section 3.1) (US Food & Drug Administration, 1976).

Total US sales of metronidazole for use in human medicine are estimated to be less than 13,000 kg annually.

It can be used as a trichomonacide in veterinary medicine (Stecher, 1968).

2.2 Occurrence

Although metronidazole is closely related to the natural antitrichomonal agent, azomycin, it is not known to occur in nature (Rollo, 1975b).

2.3 Analysis

Methods of assay of metronidazole to meet regulatory requirements for pharmaceutical products commonly employ non-aqueous titration. This has been compared to potentiometric methods for determination of metronidazole in pharmaceutical products (Tuckerman & Bican-Fister, 1969).

Bioassay procedures using agar diffusion techniques have been reported (Levison, 1974; Ralph & Kirby, 1975). Gas chromatography of the silyl derivative has been used for its determination in plasma (Midha *et al.*, 1973; Wood, 1975).

A UV spectrophotometric method for the determination of metronidazole in pharmaceutical products has been described (Kompantseva *et al.*, 1973), and colorimetric (Populaire *et al.*, 1968; Sanghavi & Chandramohan, 1974) and complexometric determinations (Gajewska, 1972) have been reported.

3. Biological Data Relevant to the Evaluation of Carcinogenic Risk to Man

3.1 Carcinogenicity and related studies in animals

Oral administration[1]

Mouse: Metronidazole was administered for lifetime in the diet of groups of 6-8-week old Swiss mice at levels of 0.06% (effective numbers: 9 males and 10 females), 0.15% (19 males and 20 females), 0.3% (18 males

---

[1]The Working Group was also aware of ongoing tests in rats (IARC, 1976).

116

and 20 females) and 0.5% (35 males and 36 females); 70 male and 70
female mice were used as untreated controls. Survival was similar in all
groups. The incidence of lung tumours rose from 19% in untreated males to
33, 58, 67 and 77% in treated males and from 20% in untreated females to
40, 50, 70 and 44% in treated females. Female mice also exhibited a significantly increased incidence of lymphomas at the two highest dose levels,
whereas no significant increase was observed in the two other groups of
treated females and in none of the groups of treated males (Rustia &
Shubik, 1972).

Rat: Metronidazole was administered at a concentration of 0.135% in
the diet to weanling female Sprague-Dawley rats for 66 weeks, followed by
a 10-week observation period; 36 rats survived for more than 10 weeks.
Twelve rats developed benign mammary fibroadenomas and 3 mammary adenocarcinomas. In an untreated control group, 12 rats developed fibroadenomas
and 6, adenocarcinomas among 71 rats surviving for more than 10 weeks.
Whereas untreated rats developed no more than one mammary tumour, those
developing mammary tumours after metronidazole treatment had an average
of 2.8 tumours per tumour-bearing rat (Cohen *et al.*, 1973).

3.2 Other relevant biological data

(a) Experimental systems

After its oral administration, metronidazole is readily absorbed from
the stomach and duodenum in rats (Populaire *et al.*, 1971). Following i.v.
administration of $(1,2-^{14}C)$-metronidazole to mice, activity was found in
liver and kidney and in heart, brain, salivary gland, gastrointestinal
tract, spleen and skeletal muscle and was shown to cross the placenta to
the foetus (Placidi *et al.*, 1970). In rats, metronidazole was conjugated
in the liver and excreted in the bile (Populaire *et al.*, 1971) and in
the urine (Mészaros & Szporny, 1968).

Metronidazole is reduced in rats by caecal flora in the absence of
oxygen (Searle & Willson, 1976) and by guinea-pig liver preparations
in vitro (Mitchard, 1971).

Metronidazole caused point mutations in *Salmonella typhimurium* TA100
without addition of liver homogenate (McCann *et al.*, 1975). It is mutagenic

only under anaerobic conditions in a mutant of TA100 that is deficient in aerobic nitroreductase activity (Rosenkranz & Speck, 1975). No mutagenic activity was found in the urine of mice treated for 4 days with daily doses of up to 400 mg/kg bw metronidazole, and marginal activity was reported in the host-mediated assay when mice were treated with 400 mg/kg bw for 5 days. S. typhimurium was used as the genetic indicator in both tests (Legator et al., 1975). In a fluctuation test, metronidazole induced streptomycin-resistant mutants in Klebsiella pneumoniae (Voogd et al., 1974).

(b) Man

Transient neutropenia was observed in 10 (3%) of 386 metronidazole-treated patients (Lefebvre & Hesseltine, 1965).

In 4 healthy male subjects given 750 mg ^{14}C-labelled metronidazole, 14% of the activity was excreted in the faeces and 77% in the urine within 5 days (Schwartz & Jeunet, 1976). In man, the major urinary metabolite is 1-(2-hydroxyethyl)-2-hydroxymethyl-5-nitroimidazole (Stambaugh et al., 1967). In addition, four other nitro-group-containing metabolites have been identified, each derived from the side-chain oxidation of the ethyl and/or methyl group. They included 1-acetic acid-2-methyl-5-nitroimidazole and 1-(2-hydroxyethyl)-2-carboxylic acid-5-nitroimidazole salt (Stambaugh et al., 1968).

In women given 250 mg metronidazole orally during pregnancy or lactation, the drug was found in low concentrations (0.25 mg/kg bw) in embryonic tissue and in milk (Amon et al., 1972).

In human patients receiving 750 mg/day, mutagenic activity was found in the urine, using Salmonella typhimurium as a genetic indicator (Legator et al., 1975). A 2-4-fold increase in the occurrence of chromosome abnormalities was observed in cultured peripheral leucocytes from patients with Crohh's disease being treated with 200-1200 mg/day metronidazole for 1-24 months (Mitelman et al., 1976).

3.3 Case reports and epidemiological studies

No data were available to the Working Group (see also 'General Remarks on Substances Considered', pp. 24-25).

4. Comments on Data Reported and Evaluation[1]

4.1 Animal data

Metronidazole is carcinogenic in mice after its oral administration: it significantly increased the incidence of lung tumours in both sexes and the incidence of lymphomas in females. Its oral administration to rats increased the incidence and multiplicity of mammary fibroadenomas.

4.2 Human data

No case reports or epidemiological studies were available to the Working Group.

---

[1]See also the section 'Animal Data in Relation to the Evaluation of Risk to Man' in the introduction to this volume, p. 13.

5. References

Amon, K., Amon, I. & Hueller, H. (1972) Maternal-fetal passage of metroni-
    dazole. In: Hejzlar, M., ed., Advances in Antimicrobiology and Anti-
    neoplastic Chemotherapy, Proceedings of International Congress of
    Chemotherapy, 7th, 1971, Baltimore, Md, University Park Press,
    pp. 113-115

Anon. (1974) Production and imports of selected drugs and pharmaceuticals
    in India. Chemical Industry News (India), July

Blacow, N.W., ed. (1972) Martindale, The Extra Pharmacopoeia, 26th ed.,
    London, Pharmaceutical Press, pp. 1095-1098

British Pharmacopoeia Commission (1973) British Pharmacopoeia, London,
    HMSO, p. 309

Carne, S. (1976) Metronidazole and acne. Lancet, ii, 367

Cohen, S.M., Ertürk, E., Van Esch, A.M., Crovetti, A.J. & Bryan, G.T.
    (1973) Carcinogenicity of 5-nitrofurans, 5-nitroimidazoles, 4-nitro-
    benzenes and related compounds. J. nat. Cancer Inst., 51, 403-417

Gajewska, M. (1972) Complexometric determination of various diazole
    derivatives with cupric picrate. Acta pol. pharm., 29, 399-404

IARC (1976) IARC Information Bulletin on the Survey of Chemicals Being
    Tested for Carcinogenicity, No. 6, Lyon, p. 244

Jacob, R.M., Régnier, G.L. & Crisan, C. (1960) Nitroimidazolealkanols and
    acyl derivatives. US Patent 2,944,061, July 5, to Société des
    usines chimiques Rhône-Poulenc

Kompantseva, E.V., Vergeichik, E.N. & Belikov, V.G. (1973) Differential
    spectrophotometric determination of metronidazole. Farmatsiya
    (Moscow), 22, 45-48

Lefebvre, Y. & Hesseltine, H.C. (1965) The peripheral white blood cells
    and metronidazole. J. Amer. med. Ass., 194, 127-130

Legator, M.S., Connor, T.H. & Stoeckel, M. (1975) Detection of mutagenic
    activity of metronidazole and niridazole in body fluids of humans and
    mice. Science, 188, 1118-1119

Levison, M.E. (1974) Microbiological agar diffusion assay for metronidazole
    concentrations in serum. Antimicrob. Agents Chemother., 5, 466-468

Mashkovski, M.D. (1972) Drug Compounds, Vol. II, Moscow, Medizina,
    pp. 390-392

McCann, J., Choi, E., Yamasaki, E. & Ames, B.N. (1975) Detection of carcinogens as mutagens in the *Salmonella*/microsome test: assay of 300 chemicals. Proc. Nat. Acad. Sci. (Wash.), 72, 5135-5139

Mészáros, C. & Szporny, L. (1968) Urinary excretion of metronidazole and isometronidazole in the rat. Acta physiol. acad. sci. hung., 34, 103-106

Midha, K.K., McGilveray, I.J. & Cooper, J.K. (1973) Determination of therapeutic levels of metronidazole in plasma by gas-liquid chromatography. J. Chromat., 87, 491-497

Mitchard, M. (1971) Bioreduction of organic nitrogen. Xenobiotica, 1, 469-481

Mitelman, F., Hartley-Asp, B. & Ursing, B. (1976) Chromosome aberrations and metronidazole. Lancet, ii, 802

Placidi, G.F., Masuoka, D., Alcaraz, A., Taylor, J.A.T. & Earle, R. (1970) Distribution and metabolism of ^{14}C-metronidazole in mice. Arch. int. Pharmacodyn., 188, 168-179

Populaire, P., Decouvelaere, B., Lebreton, G. & Pascal, S. (1968) Dosage colorimétrique de l'(hydroxy-2-éthyl)-1 méthyl-2 nitro-5 imidazole (métronidazole). Ann. pharm. franç., 26, 549-556

Populaire, P., Benazet, F., Pascal, S., Lebreton, G., Decouvelaere, B. & Guillaume, L. (1971) Circulation et sort du métronidazole dans le tractus digestif chez le rat après administration par voie orale: absorption du métronidazole par les muqueuses digestives. Thérapie, 26, 581-594

Pye, R.J. & Burton, J.L. (1976) Treatment of rosacea by metronidazole. Lancet, i, 1211-1212

Ralph, E.D. & Kirby, W.M.M. (1975) Bioassay of metronidazole with either anaerobic or aerobic incubation. J. infect. Dis., 132, 587-591

Rollo, I.M. (1975a) Drugs used in the chemotherapy of amebiasis. In: Goodman, L.S. & Gilman, A., eds, The Pharmacological Basis of Therapeutics, 5th ed., New York, Macmillan, pp. 1072-1073

Rollo, I.M. (1975b) Miscellaneous drugs used in the treatment of protozoal infections. In: Goodman, L.S. & Gilman, A., eds, The Pharmacological Basis of Therapeutics, 5th ed., New York, Macmillan, pp. 1086-1088

Rosenkranz, H.S. & Speck, W.T. (1975) Mutagenicity of metronidazole: activation by mammalian liver microsomes. Biochem. biophys. Res. Commun., 66, 520-525

Rustia, M. & Shubik, P. (1972) Induction of lung tumors and malignant lymphomas in mice by metronidazole. J. nat. Cancer Inst., 48, 721-729

Sanghavi, N.M. & Chandramohan, H.S. (1974) Methods of estimation of metronidazole. Ind. J. Pharm., 36, 151-152

Schwartz, D.E. & Jeunet, F. (1976) Comparative pharmacokinetic studies of ornidazole and metronidazole in man. Chemotherapy, 22, 19-29

Searle, A.J.F. & Willson, R.L. (1976) Metronidazole (Flagyl): degradation by the intestinal flora. Xenobiotica, 6, 457-464

Stambaugh, J.E., Feo, L.G. & Manthei, R.W. (1967) Isolation and identification of the major urinary metabolite of metronidazole. Life Sci., 6, 1811-1819

Stambaugh, J.E., Feo, L.G. & Manthei, R.W. (1968) The isolation and identification of the urinary oxidative metabolites of metronidazole in man. J. Pharmacol. exp. Ther., 161, 373-381

Stecher, P.G., ed. (1968) The Merck Index, 8th ed., Rahway, NJ, Merck & Co., p. 695

Tuckerman, M.M. & Bican-Fister, T. (1969) Analysis of metronidazole. J. pharm. Sci., 58, 1401-1403

US Food & Drug Administration (1976) Metronidazole (Flagyl) box warning. FDA Drug Bull., 6, 22-23

US International Trade Commission (1976) Synthetic Organic Chemicals, US Production and Sales, 1974, USITC Publication 776, Washington DC, US Government Printing Office, p. 101

US Pharmacopeial Convention, Inc. (1975) The US Pharmacopeia, 19th rev., Rockville, Md, pp. 327-328

US Tariff Commission (1964) Synthetic Organic Chemicals, US Production and Sales, 1963, TC Publication 143, Washington DC, US Government Printing Office, p. 134

Voogd, C.E., van der Stel, J.J. & Jacobs, J.J.J.A.A. (1974) The mutagenic action of nitroimidazoles. I. Metronidazole, nimorazole, dimetridazole and ronidazole. Mutation Res., 26, 483-490

Wood, N.F. (1975) GLC analysis of metronidazole in human plasma. J. pharm. Sci., 64, 1048-1049

NIRIDAZOLE

1. Chemical and Physical Data

1.1 Synonyms and trade names

Chem. Abstr. Reg. Serial No.: 61-57-4

Chem. Abstr. Name: 1-(5-Nitro-2-thiazolyl)-2-imidazolidinone

Nitrothiamidazol; nitrothiamidazole; nitrothiazole; 1-(5-nitro-2-thiazolyl)-2-imidazolinone; 1-(5-nitro-2-thiazolyl)-2-oxotetrahydro-imidazole

Ambilhar; 32644-Ba; Ba 32644; Ba 32644 CIBA: Ciba 32644; Ciba 32644-Ba; NTOI

1.2 Chemical formula and molecular weight

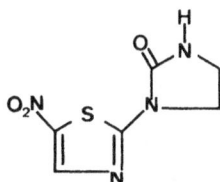

$C_6H_6N_4O_3S$ Mol. wt: 214.2

1.3 Chemical and physical properties of the pure substance

From Stecher (1968), unless otherwise specified

(a) Description: Yellow crystals from dimethylformamide

(b) Melting-point: 260-262°C

(c) Spectroscopy data: λ_{max} 370 nm (E_1^1 = 536) (Antaki & Tewfik, 1968)

1.4 Technical products and impurities

Niridazole is not commercially available in the US, but 500 mg tablets can be obtained from the Parasitic Disease Drug Service, Center for Disease Control, Atlanta, Ga (Rollo, 1975). In certain European countries, it is available in 100 mg tablets (Blacow, 1972).

2. Production, Use, Occurrence and Analysis

For important background information on this section, see preamble, p. 15.

2.1 Production and use

(a) Production

A method for the preparation of niridazole was first patented in Belgium in 1963 (Ciba Ltd, 1963). Niridazole can be prepared by the condensation of 2-chloroethyl isocyanate with 2-amino-5-nitrothiazole followed by elimination of hydrogen chloride (Archer & Yarinsky, 1972).

No evidence has been found that niridazole was ever produced commercially in the US or Japan, although Japan has imported small amounts for laboratory use. It is produced by one company in Switzerland.

(b) Use

Niridazole is effective against the three common schistosomes that may infect man, against *Entamoeba histolytica*, and against *Dracunculus medinensis* and is used clinically in all these infections. It is particularly useful in the treatment of *Schistosoma haematobium* infections but less so in infections with *S. mansoni* or *S. japonicum*. The recommended total doses for adults are 175 mg niridazole/kg bw, given orally over 5 days, for *S. haematobium* and *S. mansoni* and 100 mg/kg bw over 5 days for *S. japonicum* (WHO, 1973).

Although niridazole is an effective amoebicide, its use in the treatment of intestinal or extra-intestinal amoebiasis has largely been superceded by that of alternative drugs.

In dracontiasis, total doses of 250 mg/kg bw given over 10 days have frequently been employed.

2.2 Occurrence

Niridazole is not known to occur in nature.

2.3 Analysis

A spectrophotometric method has been used for the determination of niridazole in urine (Antaki & Tewfik, 1968). A radiochemical method employing ^{14}C-labelled niridazole was used to determine the compound and its metabolites in biological samples after their separation on a Sephadex G-25 column (Faigle & Keberle, 1969).

3. Biological Data Relevant to the Evaluation of Carcinogenic Risk to Man

3.1 Carcinogenicity and related studies in animals

Oral administration

Mouse: Administration of initial concentrations of 0.1, 0.05, 0.025 or 0% niridazole in the diet to groups of 30 male and 30 female 10-week old Swiss mice led, at the highest dose level, to significant growth retardation by 30 weeks. All groups of mice were therefore fed a basal diet for 6 weeks and were subsequently returned to diets containing niridazole at half the original concentrations. In treated mice, significantly elevated incidences of lung adenomas (37-87% *versus* 4-28% in controls) and of the number of adenomas per lung tumour-bearing mouse (3-5 *versus* 1), of carcinomas (all groups: 8 *versus* 0) and papillomas (85 *versus* 1) of the forestomach (combined: 26-63% *versus* 4%), and, in female mice, of mammary carcinomas (10-20% *versus* 4%) and ovarian granulosa-cell tumours (7-20% *versus* 0%) were observed. There were also 4 transitional-cell carcinomas of the bladder in females receiving the highest dose level and 1 in a female receiving the next highest dose level. Lymphomas were observed in treated but not in untreated male mice and in treated and untreated female mice, the latency period being reduced in treated females. The mean number of all tumours per animal was proportional to the dose given, except in the group receiving the highest dose level where survival was considerably reduced (Urman *et al.*, 1975). In a later report of the same experiment, two submucosal atypical cellular masses were found in the wall of the urinary bladder of males of the two lower dose groups and were identified as smooth-muscle tumours; these occurred after 52 and 72 weeks (Jacobs *et al.*, 1976).

Groups of at least 29 male and 29 female Swiss mice infected with 40 *Schistosoma mansoni* cercariae by Yarinsky's method (Yarinsky, 1975) and non-infected mice were fed 0.05, 0.025, 0.0125 or 0% niridazole in the diet 46 days after infection. After 25 weeks the dose levels were doubled. The incidence, distribution and latency of tumours in both infected and non-infected mice were similar to those described in the above experiment and involved lung adenomas, papillomas and carcinomas of the forestomach and bladder and carcinomas of the mammary gland and ovary (Bulay *et al.*, 1976).

Hamster: Administration of 0.24, 0.16, 0.08, 0.04 or 0% niridazole in the diet of Syrian golden hamsters either infected with 30 *Schistosoma mansoni* cercariae by Yarinsky's method (Yarinsky, 1975) 56 days before or non-infected led to a significant increase in the incidence of tumours of the forestomach, mainly papillomas, at all doses (15-90% *versus* 0-3%) except the lowest; and a total of 13 transitional-cell papillomas of the bladder were observed among animals treated with the 3 highest dose levels. The minimum numbers of animals per group were 30 males and 29 females. Infection did not appear to influence tumour yield (Bulay *et al.*, 1976).

3.2 Other relevant biological data

(a) Experimental systems

Oral administration of 0.2 or 0.4% niridazole in the diet to Swiss mice led to reduction in body weight and to severe testicular atrophy. Similar findings were observed in Syrian golden hamsters given 0.32 or 0.64% in the diet (Bulay *et al.*, 1976).

Niridazole inhibits granuloma formation and suppresses delayed hyper-sensitivity in mice (Mahmoud & Warren, 1974). It prolongs the survival of mouse skin allografts; its immunosuppressive effects have been shown to be associated with long-acting suppression of cellular immunity but not with inhibition of antibody production (Pelley *et al.*, 1975). In mice, niridazole inhibits the growth but enhances the rate of metastasis of transplanted tumours from both syngeneic and allogeneic donors (Deodhar *et al.*, 1976).

In rats, rabbits and dogs, orally administered ^{14}C-imidazinone ring-labelled niridazole is slowly but well absorbed and excreted in the urine and faeces within a few days. In experiments involving rat tissue homogenates, it was degraded most rapidly by liver and kidney and to a lesser extent by testis, spleen, heart, lung, brain, muscle and thymus - this order corresponds to the levels of nitroreductase in these tissues. Similarly, it is metabolized most rapidly *in vitro* by mouse liver and then in descending order by the liver of rats, rabbits, sheep, pigs and bovines. In blood, the metabolites attain a higher level than the parent drug (Faigle & Keberle, 1969).

The principal metabolite of niridazole formed by rat liver microsomes was the hydroxylamine (*N*-hydroxyaminothiamidazol), formed by reduction of the nitro group of niridazole (Feller *et al.*, 1971). This reduction was also mediated by rat liver xanthine oxidase (Morita *et al.*, 1971).

Mutagenicity was reported in *Salmonella typhimurium* TA100 and TA1538, in the absence of metabolic activation by liver homogenates (McCann *et al.*, 1975), and the induction of tandem duplications in *Escherichia coli* has been described (Straus, 1974). The mutagenic activity of niridazole for *Salmonella* TA1538 has also been detected in blood and urine from mice treated with 200 mg/kg bw and in the host-mediated assay after administration of 10 mg/kg bw by an unspecified route (Legator *et al.*, 1975). Mitotic recombination in *Saccharomyces cerevisiae* (D5 strain) given 100-200 µg/ml (Shahin, 1975) and specific locus mutations in the ad-3 region in *Neurospora crassa* (Ong & de Serres, 1975) have also been reported to occur. Mutagenic activity in *Salmonella typhimurium* TA1538 was detected following exposure of the bacterial test system to the urine of patients treated with 250 mg niridazole orally twice daily for ten days (Legator *et al.*, 1975).

In the dominant lethal test in mice, after either a single i.p. injection (530-650 mg/kg bw) or 5 oral doses of 125 mg/kg bw, a significant decrease in the number of pregnant animals and total implants per pregnancy, but no difference from controls in post-implantation losses, were observed (Epstein *et al.*, 1972). There is no indication of an ability to cause chromosome abnormalities after an i.p. injection of 450 mg/kg bw in bone-marrow cells of rats (Sauro & Green, 1973) or mice (Holden *et al.*, 1975). Absence of an effect on micronuclei in mouse bone-marrow cells after single i.p. injections of 10-200 mg/kg bw or multiple injections of 100 mg/kg bw for 5 days was also reported (Weber *et al.*, 1975).

(b) Man

Niridazole suppresses delayed hypersensitivity in humans (Webster
et al., 1975). Orally administered niridazole is well absorbed (Faigle &
Keberle, 1969); it is metabolized in the liver and eliminated largely
and almost equally in the urine and faeces (Rollo, 1975).

3.3 Case reports and epidemiological studies

No data were available to the Working Group (see also 'General Remarks
on Substances Considered', pp. 24-25).

4. Comments on Data Reported and Evaluation[1]

4.1 Animal data

Niridazole is carcinogenic in mice and hamsters after its oral administration: in mice it induced lymphomas and tumours of the lung, stomach,
mammary gland, ovary and bladder; in hamsters it produced tumours of the
forestomach and papillomas of the urinary bladder. Infection of treated
mice and hamsters with *Schistosoma mansoni* cercariae did not affect the
carcinogenicity of the compound.

4.2 Human data

No case reports or epidemiological studies were available to the
Working Group.

---

[1]See also the section 'Animal Data in Relation to the Evaluation of
Risk to Man' in the introduction to this volume, p. 13.

5. References

Antaki, H. & Tewfik, J. (1968) A study on the metabolism and excretion of
1-(5-nitro-2-thiazolyl)-2-imidazolidinone (nitrothiamidazole).
J. Egypt. med. Ass., 51, 991-996

Archer, S. & Yarinsky, A. (1972) Recent developements in the chemotherapy
of schistosomiasis. In: Jucker, E., ed., Progress in Drug Research,
Vol. 16, Basel, Stuttgart, Birkhäuser Verlag, pp. 14-23

Blacow, N.W., ed. (1972) Martindale, The Extra Pharmacopoeia, 26th ed.,
London, Pharmaceutical Press, pp. 1618-1621

Bulay, O., Urman, H., Clayson, D.B. & Shubik, P. (1976) Carcinogenic
effects of niridazole on rodents infected with Schistosoma mansoni.
J. nat. Cancer Inst. (in press)

Ciba Ltd (1963) New 2-oxotetrahydroimidazoles. Belgian Patent, 632,989,
29 November

Deodhar, S.D., Lee, V.W., Chiang, T., Mahmoud, A.F. & Warren, K.S. (1976)
Effects of the immunosuppressive drug niridazole in isogeneic and
allogeneic mouse tumor systems in vivo. Cancer Res., 36, 3147-3150

Epstein, S.S., Arnold, E., Andrea, J., Bass, W. & Bishop, Y. (1972)
Detection of chemical mutagens by the dominant lethal assay in the
mouse. Toxicol. appl. Pharmacol., 23, 288-325

Faigle, J.W. & Keberle, H. (1969) Metabolism of niridazole in various
species, including man. Ann. N.Y. Acad. Sci., 160, 544-557

Feller, D.R., Morita, M. & Gillette, J.R. (1971) Enzymatic reduction of
niridazole by rat liver microsomes. Biochem. Pharmacol., 20, 203-215

Holden, H.E., Ray, V.A., Wahrenburg, M.G., Ellis, J.H., Jr & Florio, J.R.
(1975) A comparative study of schistosomicides in cytogenetic and
point mutation assays. Mutation Res., 31, 309-310

Jacobs, J.B., Cohen, S.M., Arai, M., Friedell, G.H., Bulay, O. & Urman, H.K.
(1976) Chemically induced smooth muscle tumors of the mouse urinary
bladder. Cancer Res., 36, 2396-2398

Legator, M.S., Connor, T.H. & Stoeckel, M. (1975) Detection of mutagenic
activity of metronidazole and niridazole in body fluids of humans and
mice. Science, 188, 1118-1119

Mahmoud, A.A.F. & Warren, K.S. (1974) Anti-inflammatory effects of tartar
emetic and niridazole: suppression of schistosome egg granuloma.
J. Immunol., 112, 222-228

McCann, J., Choi, E., Yamasaki, E. & Ames, B.N. (1975) Detection of carcinogens as mutagens in the *Salmonella*/microsome test: assay of 300 chemcals. Proc. Nat. Acad. Sci. (Wash.), 72, 5135-5139

Morita, M., Feller, D.R. & Gillette, J.R. (1971) Reduction of niridazole by rat liver xanthine oxidase. Biochem. Pharmacol., 20, 217-226

Ong, T-M. & de Serres, F.J. (1975) Mutagenic evaluation of antischistosomal drugs and their derivatives in *Neurospora crassa*. J. Toxicol. environm. Hlth, 1, 271-279

Pelley, R.P., Pelley, R.J., Stavitsky, A.B., Mahmoud, A.A.F. & Warren, K.S. (1975) Niridazole, a potent long-acting suppressant of cellular hypersensitivity. III. Minimal suppression of antibody responses. J. Immunol., 115, 1477-1482

Rollo, I.M. (1975) Drugs used in the chemotherapy of helminthiasis. In: Goodman, L.S. & Gilman, A., eds, The Pharmacological Basis of Therapeutics, 5th ed., New York, Macmillan, pp. 1026-1027

Sauro, F.M. & Green, S. (1973) *In vivo* cytogenetic evaluation of chloroindazole thioxanthene IA-4 (a hycanthone analog) and niridazole in rat bone marrow. J. Pharmacol. exp. Ther., 186, 399-401

Shahin, M.M. (1975) Genetic activity of niridazole in yeast. Mutation Res., 30, 191-198

Stecher, P.G., ed. (1968) The Merck Index, 8th ed., Rahway, NJ, Merck & Co., pp. 733-734

Straus, D.S. (1974) Induction by mutagens of tandem gene duplications in the *glyS* region of the *Escherichia coli* chromosome. Genetics, 78, 823-830

Urman, H.K., Bulay, O., Clayson, D.B. & Shubik, P. (1975) Carcinogenic effects of niridazole. Cancer Lett., 1, 69-74

Weber, E., Bidwell, K. & Legator, M.S. (1975) An evaluation of the micronuclei test using triethylenemelamine, trimethylphosphate, hycanthone and niridazole. Mutation Res., 28, 101-106

Webster, L.T., Jr, Butterworth, A.E., Mahmoud, A.A.F., Mngola, E.N. & Warren, K.S. (1975) Suppression of delayed hypersensitivity in schistosome-infected patients by niridazole. New Engl. J. Med., 292, 1144-1147

WHO (1973) Schistosomiasis control. Wld Hlth Org. techn. Rep. Ser., No. 515, p. 18

Yarinsky, A. (1975) Evaluation of schistosomicides against experimentally established *Schistosoma mansoni* infections in mice and hamsters. J. Toxicol. environm. Hlth, 1, 229-242

1. Chemical and Physical Data

1.1 Synonyms and trade names

Chem. Abstr. Reg. Serial No.: 434-07-1

Chem. Abstr. Name: 17-Hydroxy-2-(hydroxymethylene)-17-methyl-5α,17β-androstan-3-one

4,5-Dihydro-2-hydroxymethylene-17α-methyltestosterone; HMD; 17β-hydroxy-2-hydroxymethylene-17α-methyl-3-androstanone; 17β-hydroxy-2-(hydroxymethylene)-17α-methyl-5α-androstan-3-one; 17β-hydroxy-2-(hydroxymethylene)-17-methyl-5α-androstan-3-one; 2-hydroxymethylene-17α-methyl-5α-androstan-17β-ol-3-one; 2-hydroxymethylene-17α-methyl-dihydrotestosterone; 2-(hydroxymethylene)-17-methyldihydrotesto-sterone; 2-(hydroxymethylene)-17α-methyldihydrotestosterone; 2-hydroxymethylene-17α-methyl-17β-hydroxy-3-androstanone; 17α-methyl-2-hydroxymethylene-17-hydroxy-5α-androstan-3-one; oximetholonum; oximetolona; oxymethenolone

Adroidin; Adroyd; Anadrol; Anadroyd; Anapolon; Anasteron; Anasteronal; Anasterone; Becorel; CI-406; Dynasten; Methabol; Nastenon; NSC-26 198; Oxitosona-50; Pavisoid; Plenastril; Protanabol; Roboral; Synasteron; Zenalosyn

1.2 Chemical formula and molecular weight

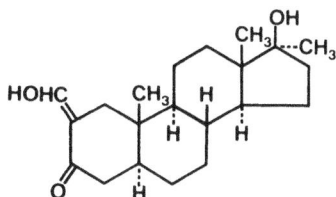

$C_{21}H_{32}O_3$ Mol. wt: 332.5

1.3 Chemical and physical properties of the pure substance

From Weast (1975), unless otherwise specified

(a) Description: Crystals (Stecher, 1968)

(b) Melting-point: 178-180°C; 182°C

(c) Optical rotation: $[\alpha]_D^{25} = +36°$ in dioxane

(d) Spectroscopy data: λ_{max} 285 and 315 nm (E_1^1 = 294 and 547) in 0.01 N methanolic sodium hydroxide

(e) Solubility: Practically insoluble in water; soluble in ethanol, dioxane and ether; very soluble in chloroform (Blacow, 1972)

1.4 Technical products and impurities

Oxymetholone is available in the US as a National Formulary grade containing 97-103% active ingredient on a dried basis with a maximum of 3% foreign steroids or other impurities. Tablets are available in 2.5, 5, 10 and 50 mg doses that contain 90-110% of the stated amount of oxymetholone (Kastrup, 1974; National Formulary Board, 1970). In Japan, oxymetholone is also available in powder form.

2. Production, Use, Occurrence and Analysis

For important background information on this section, see preamble, p. 15.

2.1 Production and use

(a) Production

A method of preparing oxymetholone was reported in 1959 and involved the following steps: 17α-methylandrostan-17β-ol-3-one in anhydrous thiophene-free benzene is reacted with ethyl formate and sodium hydride by stirring the mixture under nitrogen for several hours. The resulting sodium derivative is washed and then treated with cold dilute hydrochloric acid to liberate crude oxymetholone, which is purified by recrystallization from ethyl acetate (Ringold *et al.*, 1959).

No evidence has been found that oxymetholone was ever commercially produced in the US. In 1975, two Japanese companies produced a combined total of 480 kg oxymetholone.

132

(b) Use

Oxymetholone is a synthetic androgenic-anabolic steroid hormone primarily intended for use in clinical therapy to maintain a positive nitrogen balance. It can be used to reverse excess excretion of calcium and nitrogen resulting from corticosteroid therapy, prolonged immobilization and other diseases characterized by catabolism and tissue depletion (American Society of Hospital Pharmacists, 1968). Oxymetholone is used mainly to promote weight gain to counteract weakness and emaciation resulting from debilitating diseases and after serious infections, burns, trauma or surgery. The usual adult dosage of 5 to 10 mg per day is administered orally for about 3 weeks, but not exceeding 13 weeks, for a single course of therapy. Occasionally, 30 mg per day is given (Harvey, 1975).

Oxymetholone can also be used in the treatment of anaemias caused by deficient red-cell production and in acquired and congenital aplastic anaemias, myelofibrosis and hypoplastic anaemias due to myelotoxic drugs. It can be used as an adjunct in the treatment of senile and post-menopausal osteoporosis (Kastrup, 1974).

Total US sales of oxymetholone for use in human medicine are estimated to be less than 20 kg annually. In Japan, 360 kg are estimated to have been used in 1975.

Oxymetholone has reportedly been used in veterinary medicine as an anabolic steroid for small animals (Stecher, 1968).

2.2 Occurrence

Oxymetholone is not known to occur in nature.

2.3 Analysis

A general survey of steroid analysis includes methods for anabolic steroids (Forist & Johnson, 1961). An ultraviolet spectral assay for oxymetholone in bulk and tablet form (National Formulary Board, 1970) and thin-layer chromatographic analysis (Hara & Mibe, 1967) have been described.

3.   Biological Data Relevant to the Evaluation
of Carcinogenic Risk to Man

3.1   Carcinogenicity and related studies in animals

No data were available to the Working Group.

3.2   Other relevant biological data

(a)   Experimental systems

No data were available to the Working Group.

(b)   Man

About 5% of an oral dose of 10 mg oxymetholone was recovered from the urine as two unidentified metabolites, which were present in roughly equal proportions (Adhikary & Harkness, 1971).   Administration of oxymetholone and other androgenic anabolic agents can give rise to various alterations of liver morphology , peliosis hepatis (Bagheri & Boyer, 1974;   Bernstein *et al*., 1971;   Meadows *et al*., 1974), cholestasis and haemosiderosis (Johnson *et al*., 1972), haemorrhagic necrosis (Bruguera, 1975), haemosiderosis (Lesna *et al*., 1976) and altered liver function (Anon., 1973; Holder *et al*., 1975;   Johnson *et al*., 1972;   Mulvihill *et al*., 1975).

3.3   Case reports and epidemiological studies

Ten cases of liver-cell tumours have been reported in young patients treated with oxymetholone alone or in combination with other androgenic anabolic steroids or drugs for aplastic anaemia (5 cases), Fanconi's anaemia (3 cases) or paroxysmal nocturnal haemoglobinuria (2 cases) (see Table I). In all the cases reported, patients were treated for extended periods.   In five of these patients blood cysts (peliosis hepatis), haemorrhagic lesions or haemosiderosis were found in the neoplastic as well as in the normal tissue.   The tumours have been variously described and diagnosed owing to the difficulty of distinguishing between benign and malignant liver-cell neoplasms.   However, no metastases were demonstrated in any of the patients. In two patients the liver lesions were reported to regress after cessation of the drug (Farrell *et al*., 1975;   Johnson *et al*., 1972).

A single case of hepatocellular carcinoma was reported to have occurred in a 22-year old girl with Fanconi's anaemia diagnosed at 8 years of age

134

TABLE I

Cases of liver-cell tumours associated with oxymetholone therapy

Case no.	Age[a] (yrs)	Sex	Disease	Dose per day (mg)	Duration of treatment (months)	Other drugs	Liver function tests	α-Feto-protein	Original pathological diagnosis	Other hepatic lesions	Reference
1	20/21	M	Fanconi's anaemia	100	10	–	not reported	not tested	well-diff. hepatoma	peliosis hepatis	Bernstein et al., 1971
2[b]	2½/6½	F	aplastic anaemia	30–100	46	prednisone	normal	negative	hepatocellular carcinoma	–	Johnson et al., 1972
3	17/19½	F	aplastic anaemia	150–250	28	prednisone	abnormal	negative	well-diff. hepatocellular carcinoma	cholestasis; haemosiderosis	Johnson et al., 1972
4[c]	4/15½	M	aplastic anaemia	100	36	prednisone; methyltestosterone; norethandrolone; stanozolol	slightly abnormal	high concentration	?	?	Henderson et al., 1973
5	2/6	F	aplastic anaemia	40–60	41	prednisone; nandrolone decanoate	normal	not tested	well-diff. hepatoma	peliosis hepatis	Meadows et al., 1974
6	5/11	M	Fanconi's anaemia	not reported	13	prednisone; methandrostenolone; fluxoxymesterone; nandrolone decanoate	abnormal	negative	well-diff. hepatoma	–	Holder et al., 1975

Case no.	Age[a] (yrs)	Sex	Disease	Dose per day (mg)	Duration of treatment (months)	Other drugs	Liver function tests	α-Feto-protein	Original pathological diagnosis	Other hepatic lesions	Reference
7	16/19	M	paroxysmal nocturnal haemoglobinuria	not reported	36	–	not reported	not reported	liver-cell adenoma	haemorrhagic necrosis; blood cysts in tumour	Bruguera, 1975
8[d]	28/34	M	paroxysmal nocturnal haemoglobinuria	100–150	65	prednisone	normal	negative	well-diff. hepatocellular carcinoma	–	Farrell et al., 1975
9	8½/12	M	Fanconi's anaemia	20–200	37	prednisone	abnormal	negative	well-diff. hepatic adenoma	–	Mulvihill et al., 1975
10	2/17	M	aplastic anaemia	50	68	testosterone; prednisone; azathioprine	not reported	not tested	liver adenoma	haemosiderosis	Lesna et al., 1976

[a] Age at diagnosis of disease/age when liver tumour was diagnosed or age at death

[b] Regression of hepatic lesion shown by liver scan; death by gastrointestinal haemorrhage. No autopsy performed

[c] Diagnosis of liver tumour made on clinical basis only; oxymetholone given only during the last 3 years

[d] Decrease of liver size and regression of neoplastic lesion shown by liver scan

and not treated with androgen therapy. However, post-necrotic cirrhosis was found, which could have predisposed to development of the cancer (Cattan et al., 1974).

Eight other cases of hepatic tumours have recently been reported in patients receiving long-term therapy with other androgenic anabolic steroids for Fanconi's anaemia (5 cases), hypopituitarism (1 case), cryptorchidism (1 case) or impotence (1 case) (Corberand et al., 1975; Farrell et al., 1975; Guy & Auslander, 1973; Johnson et al., 1972; Sweeney & Evans, 1975; Ziegenfuss & Carabasi, 1973).

It has been proposed that prolonged use of such drugs may cause liver-cell damage or hyperplasia, thus prediposing to subsequent malignant transformation (Johnson et al., 1972). On the other hand, the underlying disease itself may have hepatic neoplasia as a complication, which becomes apparent when survival is extended by drugs (Committee on Neoplastic Diseases, 1974).

4. Comments on Data Reported and Evaluation

4.1 Animal data

No data were available to the Working Group.

4.2 Human data

Although ten cases of liver-cell tumours have been reported in patients with aplastic anaemia, Fanconi's anaemia or paroxysmal nocturnal haemoglobinuria treated for long periods with oxymetholone alone or in combination with other androgenic drugs, a causal relationship cannot be established.

The increased risk of developing liver-cell tumours could be related to hepatic damage known to be caused by oxymetholone. On the other hand, patients with congenital anaemias may have an intrinsically higher risk of developing tumours; this risk may become manifest during the extended survival resulting from administration of the drug.

5. References

Adhikary, P.M. & Harkness, R.A. (1971) The use of carbon skeleton chromato-graphy for the detection of steroid drug metabolites: the metabolism of anabolic steroids in man. Acta endocrinol., 67, 721-732

American Society of Hospital Pharmacists (1968) American Hospital Formulary Service, Section 68:08, Washington DC

Anon. (1973) Liver tumours and steroid hormones. Lancet, ii, 1481

Bagheri, S.A. & Boyer, J.L. (1974) Peliosis hepatis associated with andro-genic-anabolic steroid therapy. A severe form of hepatic injury. Ann. int. Med., 81, 610-618

Bernstein, M.S., Hunter, R.L. & Yachnin, S. (1971) Hepatoma and peliosis hepatis developing in a patient with Fanconi's anemia. New Engl. J. Med., 284, 1135-1136

Blacow, N.W., ed. (1972) Martindale, The Extra Pharmacopoeia, London, Pharmaceutical Press, pp. 1680-1681

Bruguera, M. (1975) Hepatoma associated with androgenic steroids. Lancet., i, 1295

Cattan, D., Kalifat, R., Wautier, J-L., Meignan, S., Vesin, P. & Piet, R. (1974) Maladie de Fanconi et cancer du foie. Arch. franç. Mal. App. dig., 63, 41-48

Committee on Neoplastic Diseases (1974) Is liver cancer induced by treating aplastic anemia with androgenic agents? Pediatrics, 53, 764

Corberand, J., Pris, J., Dutau, G., Rumeau, J-L. & Régnier, C. (1975) Association d'une maladie de Fanconi et d'une tumeur hépatique chez une malade soumise à un traitement androgénique au long cours. Arch. franç. Pédiat., 32, 275-283

Farrell, G.C., Joshua, D.E., Uren, R.F., Baird, P.J., Perkins, K.W. & Kronenberg, H. (1975) Androgen-induced hepatoma. Lancet, i, 430-432

Forist, A.A. & Johnson, J.L. (1961) Steroids. In: Higuchi, T. & Brochmann-Hanssen, E., eds, Pharmaceutical Analysis, New York, Interscience, pp. 69-136

Guy, J.T. & Auslander, M.O. (1973) Androgenic steroids and hepatocellular carcinoma. Lancet, i, 148

Hara, S. & Mibe, K. (1967) Systematic analysis of steroids. VII. Thin-layer chromatography of steroidal pharmaceuticals. Chem. pharm. Bull. (Tokyo), 15, 1036-1040

Harvey, S.C. (1975) Hormones. In: Osol, A. *et al.*, eds, Remington's Pharmaceutical Sciences, 15th ed., Easton, Pa, Mack, pp. 931-932

Henderson, J.T., Richmond, J. & Sumerling, M.D. (1973) Androgenic-anabolic steroid therapy and hepatocellular carcinoma. Lancet, i, 934

Holder, L.E., Gnarra, D.J., Lampkin, B.C., Nishiyama, H. & Perkins, P. (1975) Hepatoma associated with anabolic steroid therapy. Amer. J. Roentgenol., 124, 638-642

Johnson, F.L., Feagler, J.R., Lerner, K.G., Majerus, P.W., Siegel, M., Hartmann, J.R. & Thomas, E.D. (1972) Association of androgenic-anabolic steroid therapy with development of hepatocellular carcinoma. Lancet, ii, 1273-1276

Kastrup, E.K., ed. (1974) Facts and Comparisons, St Louis, Missouri, Facts and Comparisons, Inc., p. 111c

Lesna, M., Spencer, I. & Walker, W. (1976) Liver nodules and androgens. Lancet, i, 1124

Meadows, A.T., Naiman, J.L. & Valdes-Dapena, M. (1974) Hepatoma associated with androgen therapy for aplastic anemia. J. Pediat., 84, 109-110

Mulvihill, J.J., Ridolfi, R.L., Schultz, F.R., Borzy, M.S. & Haughton, P.B.T. (1975) Hepatic adenoma in Fanconi anemia treated with oxymetholone. J. Pediat., 87, 122-124

National Formulary Board (1970) National Formulary XIII, Washington DC, American Pharmaceutical Association, pp. 506-508

Ringold, H.J., Batres, E., Halpern, O. & Necoechea, E. (1959) Steroids. CV. 2-Methyl and 2-hydroxymethylene-androstane derivatives. J. Amer. chem. Soc., 81, 427-432

Stecher, P.G., ed. (1968) The Merck Index, 8th ed., Rahway, NJ, Merck & Co., p. 775

Sweeney, E.C. & Evans, D.J. (1975) Liver lesions and androgenic steroid therapy. Lancet, ii, 1042

Weast, R.C., ed. (1975) CRC Handbook of Chemistry and Physics, 56th ed., Cleveland, Ohio, Chemical Rubber Co., p. C-752

Ziegenfuss, J. & Carabasi, R. (1973) Androgens and hepatocellular carcinoma. Lancet, i, 262

PHENACETIN

1. Chemical and Physical Data

1.1 Synonyms and trade names[1]

Chem. Abstr. Reg. Serial No.: 62-44-2

Chem. Abstr. Name: *N*-(4-Ethoxyphenyl)acetamide

para-Acetophenetide; *para*-acetophenetidide; acetophenetidin; acetophenetidine; *para*-acetophenetidine; aceto-4-phenetidine; acetophenetin; acet*para*phenalide; acetphenetidin; *para*-acetphenetidin; acet-*para*-phenetidin; *N*-acetyl-*para*-phenetidine; 4'-ethoxyacetanilide; 4-ethoxyacetanilide; *para*-ethoxyacetanilide; *para*-phenacetin; phenacetine; phenacitin; phenazetin

Fenacetina; Fenedina; Fenidina; Fenina; Pertonal; Phenacet; Phenacetinum; Phenazetin; Phenedina; Phenidin; Phenin

1.2 Chemical formula and molecular weight

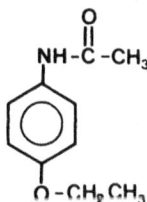

$C_{10}H_{13}NO_2$ Mol. wt: 179.2

1.3 Chemical and physical properties of the pure substance

From Stecher (1968), unless otherwise specified

(a) Description: Crystalline scales or powder

(b) Melting-point: 134-135°C

---

[1]Only trade names of those products that contain phenacetin alone are given; there are many other products in which phenacetin is combined with other drugs.

(c) Spectroscopy data: λ_{max} 250 nm in ethanol (US Pharmacopeial
Convention, Inc., 1970); 285 nm in chloroform and isooctane
(National Formulary Board, 1970)

(d) Solubility: Soluble in cold water (0.076 g/100 ml), in boiling
water (1.2 g/100 ml), in ethanol (6.7 g/100 ml), in chloroform
(7.1 g/100 ml), in ether (1.1 g/100 ml) and in glycerol

1.4 Technical products and impurities

Various national and international pharmacopoeias give specifications
for the purity of phenacetin in pharmaceutical products. For example,
phenacetin is available in the US as a USP grade containing 98-101%
active ingredient on a dried basis and 0.03% maximum *para*-chloroacetanilide;
it is also obtainable as tablets in 300 mg doses containing 94-106% of
the stated amount (US Pharmacopeial Convention, Inc., 1970). Phenacetin is
also available in the US in tablet form containing 150 mg phenacetin in
combination with 230 mg aspirin and 15 or 30 mg caffeine, or with 230 mg
aspirin, 30 mg caffeine and 8, 15, 30 or 60 mg codeine phosphate and
containing 90-110% of the stated amount of phenacetin (National Formulary
Board, 1970).

2. Production, Use, Occurrence and Analysis

For important background information on this section, see preamble,
p. 15.

2.1 Production and use

(a) Production

A method of preparing phenacetin was first reported in 1894 and
involved reaction of 4-acetaminophenol with potassium ethyl sulphate in an
aqueous alcoholic alkaline solution under pressure at 150°C (Prager &
Jacobson, 1930). Phenacetin can also be prepared by condensing *para*-
nitrophenol, dissolved in a sodium hydroxide solution, with ethyl bromide
to give *para*-nitrophenetole, which is then reduced with sodium sulphide.
The resulting *para*-phenetidine is acetylated by refluxing with acetic
anhydride to give phenacetin (Swinyard, 1975).

142

In Japan, phenacetin is produced commercially by the phenol synthesis process, which uses the following materials: *para*-nitrophenol, sodium nitrate, sulphuric acid and ethyl iodide, or by the nitration-fractional crystallization process, which uses *para*-chloronitrobenzene and mixed acid.

Phenacetin has been produced commercially in the US for over 50 years (US Tariff Commission, 1927); only one US company reported production (see preamble, p. 15) in 1974 (US International Trade Commission, 1976a). The combined production of the acetanilide derivatives, phenacetin and acetaminophen, was reported to be 3,500 thousand kg in 1974 (US International Trade Commission, 1976a). US imports of phenacetin through the principal customs districts were 67,000 kg in 1972 (US Tariff Commission, 1973), 94,000 kg in 1973 (US Tariff Commission, 1974) and 192,000 kg in 1974 (US International Trade Commission, 1976b).

Phenacetin was first produced in Japan in 1935. Two companies manufactured a combined total of 276,000 kg in 1975; in that year, 40,000 kg were imported from France and less than 1,000 kg exported.

Total annual production of phenacetin in western Europe is estimated to be 1-5 million kg; the Federal Republic of Germany and France are believed to be major producing countries.

(b) Use

Phenacetin is used as an analgesic and antipyretic agent but has little anti-inflammatory activity. It is used mainly to counteract mild to moderate pain of the musculoskeletal system and is frequently combined with aspirin and caffeine. The usual dosage is 300 mg taken 4 to 6 times per day, not exceeding 2 g per day (Swinyard, 1975). Preparations containing phenacetin combined with other drugs usually contain 150 to 200 mg phenacetin (American Society of Hospital Pharmacists, 1959).

Total US sales of phenacetin for use in human medicine are estimated to be less than 640,000 kg annually.

Phenacetin is also used as a stabilizer for hydrogen peroxide in hair bleaching preparations (Markland, 1966). In veterinary medicine, it is used as an analgesic and antipyretic agent (Stecher, 1968).

2.2 Occurrence

Phenacetin is not known to occur in nature.

2.3 Analysis

Methods of assay for phenacetin that meet regulatory requirements for pharmaceutical products include non-aqueous titration, gravimetric methods and UV spectrophotometry. A selective UV spectrophotometric method based on measurement of its oxidation products by cobaltic oxide can determine phenacetin in biological materials in the range of 5-50 μg/ml (Wallace *et al.*, 1973).

A gas chromatographic method can determine phenacetin in mixtures with other drugs (Ryabtseva *et al.*, 1970), and another determines phenacetin in urine and plasma (after its conversion to a silyl derivative) with a limit of detection of 0.05 μg/ml (Prescott, 1971).

Colorimetric methods include a determination of phenacetin in formulations with aspirin and codeine phosphate (Wosiak & Krzemińska, 1975), an assay for phenacetin based on its reaction with 1,2-naphthoquinone-4-sulphonate (Nomura *et al.*, 1966) and a procedure based on oxidation of phenacetin with cerium (St. Ajer *et al.*, 1969).

3. Biological Data Relevant to the Evaluation of Carcinogenic Risk to Man

3.1 Carcinogenicity and related studies in animals

Oral administration

Rat: A group of 30 BD rats, 100 days of age (sex unspecified), received 40-50 mg/animal phenacetin daily in the diet (average total dose, 22 g). One rat died after a total dose of 10 g and was found to have an osteochondroma. The mean age at death was 770 days, compared with 750 days in an unspecified number of controls. No tumours related to treatment were observed (Schmähl & Reiter, 1954).

Four groups of 15, 20, 20 and 24 male albino rats (150-180 g) were fed diets containing 0 (control), 0.05, 0.1 or 0.5% N-hydroxyphenacetin (a putative metabolite of phenacetin) for up to 73 weeks. Of treated

144

animals 11, 13 and 15 rats were still alive at the time of the appearance
of the first tumour after 45, 45 and 38 weeks, and 8/11, 13/13 and 15/15
developed liver tumours (described as hepatocellular carcinomas), compared
with 0/15 controls; one animal fed 0.1% in the diet developed a transitional-
cell carcinoma of the renal pelvis (Calder *et al.*, 1976).

3.2 Other relevant biological data

(a) Experimental systems

The single oral LD_{50} of phenacetin in male Wistar rats is about 4 g/
kg bw (Boyd & Hottenroth, 1968) and in guinea-pigs 2.6 g/kg bw (Boyd &
Carro-Ciampi, 1970).

Papillary necrosis of the kidney was produced in Wistar rats fed a
mixture of aspirin (210 mg/kg bw/day), phenacetin (210 mg/kg bw/day) and
caffeine (80 mg/kg bw/day) but not in rats receiving 500 mg/kg bw/day
phenacetin alone (Saker & Kincaid-Smith, 1969).

There are three known metabolic pathways for phenacetin: de-ethylation,
N-deacetylation and ring hydroxylation. The main route is oxidative de-
ethylation, giving rise to *N*-acetyl-*para*-aminophenol, which is excreted in
the urine as the sulphate or as the glucuronide (Dubach & Raaflaub, 1969).
In rats, rabbits, guinea-pigs and ferrets given 125 mg/kg bw by oral intu-
bation or mixed with food, 63, 57, 81 and 47% of the dose, respectively,
were excreted as *N*-acetyl-*para*-aminophenol (free or conjugated). Metabolism
by the second pathway, N-deacetylation, was greatest in rats (21% of the
dose) and least in guinea-pigs and rabbits (7 and 4% of the dose) (Smith
& Timbrell, 1974). The *para*-phenetidine resulting from N-deacetylation
can be converted to 2-hydroxy-*para*-phenetidine, which in rats is excreted
in increasing amounts with increasing doses of phenacetin (Dubach &
Raaflaub, 1969). Other metabolites that have been found in the urine of
rats, guinea-pigs and rabbits are 2-hydroxyphenacetin and 3[(5-acetamido-2-
hydroxyphenyl)thio]aniline (Smith & Timbrell, 1974); and the 2-hydroxy-
acetophenetidine-glucuronide conjugate has been found in the urine of dogs
and cats administered phenacetin (route not given) (Klutch *et al.*, 1966).

The possible role of N-hydroxylation in the metabolism of phenacetin
has been discussed by Nery (1971). *N*-Hydroxyphenacetin, a synthetic

compound, under acid conditions or after N-ester formation, will react with methionine to give 4-hydroxy-3-methylthioacetanilide (Calder *et al.*, 1974), a urinary metabolite of phenacetin in dogs (Focella *et al.*, 1972).

In rats treated with 3-methylcholanthrene or exposed to cigarette smoke (which caused the induction of benzo[*a*]pyrene hydroxylase in lung tissue), there was an increased ability of lung and intestine to metabolize phenacetin to *N*-acetyl-*para*-aminophenol (Welch *et al.*, 1972).

A comparison of the metabolism of phenacetin with that of other structurally-related compounds has been made in rats (Smith & Griffiths, 1976).

N-Hydroxy derivatives of phenacetin were found to be nephrotoxic in female Wistar rats following single i.v. injections of about 1 mM/kg bw (Calder *et al.*, 1973).

In a limited study, an intragastric dose of 2 g/kg bw/week (equivalent to a human dose of about 20 g/day) was given in five divided doses/week to 25 male rats for up to 220 days; at 176 days 80% of the rats were sterile. No significant difference in the number of stillborns was seen compared to that in controls (Boyd, 1971).

Phenacetin can be N-nitrosated *in vitro* to form an unstable N-nitroso compound, *N*-nitroso-2-nitro-4-ethoxyacetanilide (Eisenbrand & Preussmann, 1975).

(b) Man

The main toxic effect of chronic phenacetin ingestion is papillary necrosis of the kidney (see section 3.3). Several acute cases of poisoning with paracetamol (a major metabolite of phenacetin) have been reported, in which hepatic damage occurred (Clark *et al.*, 1973; Prescott *et al.*, 1971; Proudfoot & Wright, 1970).

A group of 623 women known regularly to ingest phenacetin-containing analgesics were compared over a 4-year period with a group of 621 controls. A high intake of phenacetin analgesics was associated with increased serum creatinine levels and a low urine specific gravity (Dubach *et al.*, 1975).

Methaemoglobinaemia and haemolytic anaemia have occurred in subjects ingesting phenacetin; methaemoglobinaemia has been associated with the excretion of increased amounts of 2-hydroxyphenetidine sulphate and the glucuronide or its oxidation products in the urine of these subjects (Shahidi, 1967; Shahidi & Hemaidan, 1969; Woodbury & Fingl, 1975).

Normal subjects ingesting phenacetin excrete the major part of the dose in the urine as conjugated N-acetyl-para-aminophenol (about 70-80%), some as free N-acetyl-para-aminophenol (3-5%), a small percentage (0.2%) as unchanged phenacetin and a smaller percentage (0.1%) as para-phenetidine (Brodie & Axelrod, 1949). In 3 male volunteers given 2 g phenacetin orally, about 2% of the dose was found to be excreted as S-(1-acetamido-4-hydroxy-phenyl)cysteine in the urine (Jagenburg & Toczko, 1964). In cigarette smokers, there is a higher ratio of N-acetyl-para-aminophenol:phenacetin in the plasma than in corresponding controls (Pantuck et al., 1974).

The urinary excretion of 2-hydroxyphenetidin and of N-acetyl-para-aminophenol, and of their conjugates, was significantly decreased when phenacetin was ingested in combination with aspirin, caffeine and codeine (Gault et al., 1972).

3.3 Case reports and epidemiological studies

(a) Case reports

Hultengren et al. (1965) in Stockholm, Sweden, reported 6 cases of renal papillary necrosis associated with transitional-cell carcinoma of the renal pelvis; 5 of the cases were reported to be heavy users of phenacetin-containing analgesics (more than 1 g analgesic per day for more than one year). Since that time there have been several case reports of carcinomas of the renal pelvis (RP) or of the bladder (B) in heavy users of phenacetin-containing analgesics (Adam et al., 1970, 1 case RP; Begley et al., 1970, 1 case B; Grob, 1971, 2 cases RP; Güller & Dubach, 1973, 1 case RP, 1 case B; Liu et al., 1972, 1 case RP; Mannion & Susmano, 1971, 1 case B; Rathert et al., 1975, 1 case RP, 1 case B).

(b) Epidemiological studies

Of 242 patients in Göteborg, Sweden, with chronic non-obstructive pyelonephritis, 142 were considered to be heavy users of phenacetin-containing analgesics; 104 of these cases were followed for 1-11 years (average 5.3 years) and compared with 88 control cases not considered to be heavy users of analgesics. Eight patients in the heavy users' group developed transitional-cell carcinomas of the renal pelvis; in seven, a renal papillary necrosis was present. In addition, one male and one female developed similar tumours of the bladder. No such tumours were observed in the control group (Bengtsson *et al.*, 1968). A ninth patient later developed renal pelvic carcinoma (Angervall *et al.*, 1969).

In another report from Jönköping County Hospital, Sweden, 15 cases of transitional-cell carcinoma of the renal pelvis were observed during a 9-year period: 10 cases occurred among the inhabitants of Huskvarna (population 13,000), and 9 of these were among the workers of a small-arms factory employing 1800 people. This compares with an incidence of renal pelvic carcinoma or papilloma in Sweden as a whole of only 1 case per 183,000 per year during 1960-1963. In 10 (or possibly 12) cases, heavy use of Hjorton's powder (each dose containing 0.5 g phenacetin, 0.5 g phenazone and 0.15 g caffeine) was recorded, and renal papillary necrosis was present in 9 (or possibly 10) cases. Two of the heavy users also had a carcinoma of the bladder. The study did not include a careful search for other possible carcinogenic agents, but, according to the authors, an occupational carcinogen seemed unlikely in a factory of this type (manufacturing small-arms, sewing machines, bicycles, garden tools and similar products) (Angervall *et al.*, 1969).

In a further report of 62 cases of carcinoma of the renal pelvis in known phenacetin users (which included 19 of the cases described in the two previous reports), detailed data on the use of phenacetin-containing analgesics were available for 38 cases reported. The average total dose was 9.1 kg, average exposure time, 17 years and average induction time, 22 years. Papillary necrosis was a prominent feature in 59 patients; 8 patients also had urinary bladder tumours (Bengtsson *et al.*, 1975; Johansson *et al.*, 1974).

Bock & Hogrefe (1972) described 31 cases in the Federal Republic of Germany of carcinoma of the renal pelvis, 5 carcinomas of the ureter and 106 carcinomas of the bladder; only 1 case of papillary carcinoma of the renal pelvis associated with a benign papilloma of the ureter and 2 cases of carcinoma of the bladder were found in heavy users of phenacetin.

Taylor (1972) reported that in the UK in a series of 189 primary tumours of the adult urinary tract, 2/30 carcinomas of the renal body, 7/13 carcinomas of the renal pelvis, 0/2 carcinomas of the ureter and 2/144 carcinomas of the bladder occurred in people making heavy use of analgesics, including phenacetin-containing mixtures.

In a survey in Zurich, Switzerland, of 24,683 autopsies, 5/269 hyper-nephroid carcinomas (1.9%), 4/15 carcinomas of the renal pelvis (26.6%) and 11/218 carcinomas of the bladder (5%) were found in heavy users of phenacetin-containing analgesics. Papillary necrosis was present in 9 of these 20 subjects. Only the carcinomas of the renal pelvis were considered to be related to heavy use of phenacetin (Küng, 1976).

Of 320 patients in Denmark with a diagnosis of chronic pyelonephritis, 101 had a history of heavy use of phenacetin-containing analgesics; 2 of these presented papillary necrosis and a transitional-cell tumour of the renal pelvis (Høybye & Nielsen, 1971). Leistenschneider & Ehmann (1973) in Basel, Switzerland, reported that of 17 cancers of the renal pelvis (out of 21,291 autopsies), 8 occurred in heavy users of phenacetin-containing analgesics (2 presented pyelonephritis).

In a case-control study in the UK, in which subjects with urinary-tract cancer were compared with age and sex-matched controls, heavy consumption of analgesics was not found to be associated with cancers of the renal pelvis but was associated with cancers of the renal parenchyma. In 106 patients with adenocarcinomas of the renal parenchyma there were 15 heavy users of analgesics, and only 2 in 106 controls. It must be noted that only 4 of the 15 heavy users with a renal parenchymal tumour were users of analgesic mixtures containing phenacetin (Armstrong *et al.*, 1976).

4. Comments on Data Reported and Evaluation

4.1 Animal data

In one limited study in which phenacetin was administered orally to rats, no carcinogenic effects were observed[1]. One putative metabolite of phenacetin, *N*-hydroxyphenacetin, is carcinogenic in rats after its oral administration: it produced hepatocellular carcinomas.

4.2 Human data

Available data indicate that heavy use of analgesic mixtures containing phenacetin is associated with papillary necrosis of the kidney and suggest a relationship between such use and the development of transitional-cell carcinoma of the renal pelvis.

---

[1]The Working Group was aware that several studies on the carcinogenicity of phenacetin are underway (IARC, 1976).

5. References

Adam, W.R., Dawborn, J.K., Price, C.G., Riddell, J. & Story, H. (1970) Anaplastic transitional-cell carcinoma of the renal pelvis in association with analgesic abuse. Med. J. Austr., 1, 1108-1109

American Society of Hospital Pharmacists (1959) American Hospital Formulary Service, Section 28:08, Washington DC

Angervall, L., Bengtsson, U., Zetterlund, C.G. & Zsigmond, M. (1969) Renal pelvic carcinoma in a Swedish district with abuse of a phenacetin-containing drug. Brit. J. Urol., 41, 401-405

Armstrong, B., Garrod, A. & Doll, R. (1976) A retrospective study of renal cancer with special reference to coffee and animal protein consumption. Brit. J. Cancer, 33, 127-136

Begley, M., Chadwick, J.M. & Jepson, R.P. (1970) A possible case of analgesic abuse associated with transitional-cell carcinoma of the bladder. Med. J. Austr., 2, 1133-1134

Bengtsson, U., Angervall, L., Ekman, H. & Lehmann, L. (1968) Transitional cell tumors of the renal pelvis in analgesic abusers. Scand. J. Urol. Nephrol., 2, 145-150

Bengtsson, U., Angervall, L., Johansson, S. & Wahlgvist, L. (1975) Phenacetin abuse and renal pelvic carcinoma. Int. J. clin. Pharmacol., 12, 290-294

Bock, K.D. & Hogrefe, J. (1972) Analgetika-Abusus und maligne Tumoren der ableitenden Harnwege - Eine retrospektive Studie. Münch. med. Wschr., 114, 645-652

Boyd, E.M. (1971) Sterility from phenacetin. J. clin. Pharmacol., 11, 96-102

Boyd, E.M. & Carro-Ciampi, G. (1970) The oral 100-day LD_{50} index of phenacetin in guinea pigs. Toxicol. appl. Pharmacol., 16, 232-238

Boyd, E.M. & Hottenroth, S.M.H. (1968) The toxicity of phenacetin at the range of the oral LD_{50} (100 days) in albino rats. Toxicol. appl. Pharmacol., 12, 80-93

Brodie, B.B. & Axelrod, J. (1949) The fate of acetophenetidin (phenacetin) in man and methods for the estimation of acetophenetidin and its metabolites in biological material. J. Pharmacol. exp. Ther., 97, 58-67

Calder, I.C., Creek, M.J., Williams, P.J., Funder, C.C., Green, C.R., Ham, K.N. & Tange, J.D. (1973) N-Hydroxylation of p-acetophenetidide as a factor in nephrotoxicity. J. med. Chem., 16, 499-502

Calder, I.C., Creek, M.J. & Williams, P.J. (1974) N-Hydroxyphenacetin as a precursor of 3-substituted 4-hydroxyacetanilide metabolites of phenacetin. Chem.-biol. Interact., 8, 87-90

Calder, I.C., Goss, D.E., Williams, P.J., Funder, C.C., Green, C.R., Ham, K.N. & Tange, J.D. (1976) Neoplasia in the rat induced by N-hydroxy-phenacetin, a metabolite of phenacetin. Pathology, 8, 1-6

Clark, R., Thompson, R.P.H., Borirakchanyavat, V., Widdop, B., Davidson, A.R., Goulding, R. & Williams, R. (1973) Hepatic damage and death from over-dose of paracetamol. Lancet, i, 66-70

Dubach, U.C. & Raaflaub, J. (1969) Neue Aspekte zur Frage der Nephro-toxizität von Phenacetin. Experientia, 25, 956-958

Dubach, U.C., Levy, P.S., Rosner, B., Baumeler, H.R., Müller, A., Peier, A. & Ehrensperger, T. (1975) Relation between regular intake of phena-cetin-containing analgesics and laboratory evidence for urorenal dis-orders in a working female population of Switzerland. Lancet, i, 539-543

Eisenbrand, G. & Preussmann, R. (1975) Nitrosation of phenacetin. Formation of N-nitroso-2-nitro-4-ethoxyacetanilide as an unstable product of the nitrosation in dilute aqueous-acidic solution. Arzneimittel-Forsch., 25, 1472-1475

Focella, A., Heslin, P. & Teitel, S. (1972) The synthesis of two phenacetin metabolites. Canad. J. Chem., 50, 2025-2030

Gault, M.H., Shahidi, N.T. & Gabe, A. (1972) The effect of acetylsalicylic acid, caffeine, and codeine on the excretion of phenacetin metabolites. Canad. J. Physiol. Pharmacol., 50, 809-816

Grob, H.U. (1971) Phenazetinabusus und Nierenbeckenkarzinom. Helv. chir. acta, 38, 537-539

Güller, R. & Dubach, U.C. (1973) Tumoren der Harnwege nach regelmässiger Einnahme phenazetinhaltiger Analgetika? Helv. med. acta, 36, 247-250

Høybye, G. & Nielsen, O.E. (1971) Renal pelvic carcinoma in phenacetin abusers. Scand. J. Urol. Nephrol., 5, 190-192

Hultengren, N., Lagergren, C. & Ljungqvist, A. (1965) Carcinoma of the renal pelvis in renal papillary necrosis. Acta chir. scand., 130, 314-320

IARC (1976) IARC Information Bulletin on the Survey of Chemicals Being Tested for Carcinogenicity, No. 6, Lyon, pp. 71, 91, 279

Jagenburg, O.R. & Toczko, K. (1964) The metabolism of acetophenetidine. Isolation and characterization of S-(1-acetamido-4-hydroxyphenyl)-cysteine, a metabolite of acetophenetidine. Biochem. J., 92, 639-643

Johansson, S., Angervall, L., Bengtsson, U. & Wahlqvist, L. (1974) Uroepithelial tumors of the renal pelvis associated with abuse of phenacetin-containing analgesics. Cancer, 33, 743-753

Klutch, A., Harfenist, M. & Conney, A.H. (1966) 2-Hydroxyacetophenetidine, a new metabolite of acetophenetidine. J. med. Chem., 9, 63-66

Küng, L.G. (1976) Hypernephroides Karzinom und Karzinome der ableitenden Harnwege nach Phenacetinabusus. Schweiz. med. Wschr., 106, 47-51

Leistenschneider, W. & Ehmann, R. (1973) Nierenbeckenkarzinom nach Phenazetinabusus. Schweiz. med. Wschr., 103, 433-439

Liu, T., Smith, G.W. & Rankin, J.T. (1972) Renal pelvic tumour associated with analgesic abuse. Canad. med. Ass. J., 107, 768, 771

Mannion, R.A. & Susmano, D. (1971) Phenacetin abuse causing bladder tumor. J. Urol., 106, 692

Markland, W.R. (1966) Hair preparations. In: Kirk, R.E. & Othmer, D.F., eds, Encyclopedia of Chemical Technology, 2nd ed., Vol. 10, New York, John Wiley and Sons, pp. 798-799

National Formulary Board (1970) National Formulary XIII, Washington DC, American Pharmaceutical Association, pp. 66-68 & 178-180

Nery, R. (1971) The possible role of N-hydroxylation in the biological effects of phenacetin. Xenobiotica, 1, 339-343

Nomura, N., Ito, T. & Shiho, D. (1966) Determination of mixed medicines I. Quantitative colorimetric method for phenacetin with sodium 1,2-naphthoquinone-4-sulfonate. Yakugaku Zasshi, 86, 331-335

Pantuck, E.J., Hsiao, K-C., Maggio, A., Nakamura, K., Kuntzman, R. & Conney, A.H. (1974) Effect of cigarette smoking on phenacetin metabolism. Clin. Pharmacol. Ther., 15, 9-17

Prager, B. & Jacobson, P., eds (1930) Beilsteins Handbuch der Organischen Chemie, 4th ed., Vol. 13, Syst. 1847, Berlin, Springer-Verlag, p. 461

Prescott, L.F. (1971) The gas-liquid chromatographic estimation of phenacetin and paracetamol in plasma and urine. J. Pharm. Pharmacol., 23, 111-115

Prescott, L.F., Wright, N., Roscoe, P. & Brown, S.S. (1971) Plasma-paracetamol half-life and hepatic necrosis in patients with paracetamol overdosage. Lancet, i, 519-522

Proudfoot, A.T. & Wright, N. (1970) Acute paracetamol poisoning. Brit. med J., iii, 557-558

Rathert, P., Melchior, H. & Lutzeyer, W. (1975) Phenacetin: a carcinogen for the urinary tract? J. Urol., 133, 653-657

Ryabtseva, I.M., Kuleshova, M.I., Rudenko, B.A. & Kucherov, V.F. (1970) Gas-liquid chromatography of drugs. Izv. Akad. Nauk SSR, Ser. Khim., 12, 2676-2680

Saker, B.M. & Kincaid-Smith, P. (1969) Papillary necrosis in experimental analgesic nephropathy. Brit. med. J., i, 161-162

Schmähl, D. & Reiter, A. (1954) Fehlen einer cancerogenen Wirkung beim Phenacetin. Arzneimittel-forsch., 4, 404-405

Shahidi, N.T. (1967) Acetophenetidin sensitivity. Amer. J. Dis. Child., 113, 81-82

Shahidi, N.T. & Hemaidan, A. (1969) Acetophenetidin-induced methemoglobinemia and its relation to the excretion of diazotizable amines. J. Lab. clin. Med., 74, 581-585

Smith, G.E. & Griffiths, L.A. (1976) Comparative metabolic studies of phenacetin and structurally-related compounds in the rat. Xenobiotica, 6, 217-236

Smith, R.L. & Timbrell, J.A. (1974) Factors affecting the metabolism of phenacetin. I. Influence of dose, chronic dosage, route of administration and species on the metabolism of $[1-^{14}C-acetyl]$phenacetin. Xenobiotica, 4, 489-501

St. Ajer, G., Laszl, O.V. & Szab, O.A.E. (1969) Cerimetric determination of phenacetin. Acta pharm. hung., 39, 237-240

Stecher, P.G., ed. (1968) The Merck Index, 8th ed., Rahway, NJ, Merck & Co., p. 8

Swinyard, E.A. (1975) Analgesics and antipyretics. In: Osol, A. et al., eds, Remington's Pharmaceutical Sciences, 15th ed., Easton, Pa, Mack, p. 1051

Taylor, J.S. (1972) Carcinoma of the urinary tract and analgesic abuse. Med. J. Austr., 1, 407-409

US International Trade Commission (1976a) Synthetic Organic Chemicals, US Production and Sales, 1974, USITC Publication 776, Washington DC, US Government Printing Office, pp. 96 and 104

US International Trade Commission (1976b) Imports of Benzenoid Chemicals and Products, 1974, USITC Publication 762, Washington DC, US Government Printing Office, p. 85

US Pharmacopeial Convention, Inc. (1970) The US Pharmacopeia, 18th rev., Bethesda, Md, pp. 483-485

US Tariff Commission (1927) Census of Dyes and Other Synthetic Organic Chemicals, 1926, Tariff Information Series No. 35, Washington DC, US Government Printing Office, p. 70

US Tariff Commission (1973) Imports of Benzenoid Chemicals and Products, 1972, TC Publication 601, Washington DC, US Government Printing Office, p. 87

US Tariff Commission (1974) Imports of Benzenoid Chemicals and Products, 1973, TC Publication 688, Washington DC, US Government Printing Office, p. 83

Wallace, J.E., Biggs, J.D., Hamilton, H.E., Foster, L.L. & Blum, K. (1973) UV spectrophotometric method for determination of phenacetin in biological specimens. J. pharm. Sci., 62, 599-601

Welch, R.M., Cavallito, J. & Loh, A. (1972) Effect of exposure to cigarette smoke on the metabolism of benzo[a]pyrene and acetophenetidin by lung and intestine of rats. Toxicol. appl. Pharmacol., 23, 749-758

Woodbury, D.M. & Fingl, E. (1975) Analgesic-antipyretics, anti-inflammatory agents, and drugs employed in the therapy of gout. In: Goodman, L.S. & Gilman, A., eds, The Pharmacological Basis of Therapeutics, 5th ed., New York, Macmillan, pp. 343-347

Wosiak, B. & Krzemińska, A. (1975) Colorimetric determination of phenacetin in powders also containing aspirin and codeine phosphate. Farm. pol., 31, 771-773

PHENOBARBITAL AND PHENOBARBITAL SODIUM

1. Chemical and Physical Data

Phenobarbital

1.1 Synonyms and trade names

Chem. Abstr. Reg. Serial No.: 50-06-6

Chem. Abstr. Name: 5-Ethyl-5-phenyl-2,4,6-($1H$,$3H$,$5H$)pyrimidinetrione

5-Ethyl-5-phenylbarbituric acid; phenobarbitone; phenobarbituric acid; phenylbarbital; phenylethylbarbiturate; phenylethylbarbituric acid; 5-phenyl-5-ethylbarbituric acid; phenylethylmalonylurea

Adonal; Aephenal; Agrypnal; Amylofene; Aphenylbarbit; Aphenyletten; Austrominal; Barbapil; Barbellen; Barbellon; Barbenyl; Barbilettae; Barbinal; Barbiphen; Barbiphenyl; Barbipil; Barbita; Barbivis; Barbonal; Barbophen; Bardorm; Bartol; Bialminal; Blu-phen; Cabronal; Calmetten; Calminal; Cardenal; Cemalonal; Codibarbital; Coronaletta; Damoral; Dezibarbitur; Dormina; Dormiral; Doscalun; Duneryl; Ensobarb; Ensodorm; Epanal; Epidorm; Epilol; Episedal; Epsylone; Eskabarb; Etilfen; Euneryl; Fenbital; Fenemal; Feno-barbital; Fenosed; Fenylettae; Gardenal; Gardepanyl; Glysoletten; Haplopan; Haplos; Helional; Hennoletten; Hypnaletten; Hypnogen; Hypnolone; Hypno-Tablinetten; Hypnotal; Hysteps; Lefebar; Leonal; Lephebar; Lepinal; Linasen; Liquital; Lixophen; Lubergal; Lubrokol; Lumen; Lumesettes; Lumesyn; Luminal; Lumofridetten; Luphenil; Luramin; Molinal; Neurobarb; Nirvonal; Noptil; Nova-Pheno; Numol; Nunol; Parkotal; PEBA; Pharmetten; Phenaemal; Phen-Bar; Phenemal; Phenobal; Phenobarbyl; Phenoluric; Phenonyl; Phenoturic; Phenyletten; Phenyral; Phob; Polcominal; Promptonal; Sedabar; Seda-Tablinen; Sedicat; Sedizorin; Sedlyn; Sedofen; Sedonal; Sedonettes; Sevenal; Sombutol; Somnolens; Somnoletten; Somnosan; Somonal; Spasepilin; Starifen; Starilettae; Stental Extentabs; Teolaxin; Thenobarbital; Triabarb; Tridezibarbitur; Triphenatol; Versomnal; Zadoletten; Zadonal

1.2 Chemical formula and molecular weight

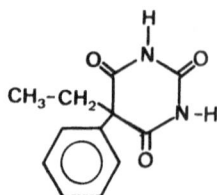

$$C_{12}H_{12}N_2O_3 \qquad \text{Mol. wt: } 232.2$$

1.3 Chemical and physical properties of the pure substance

From Stecher (1968), unless otherwise specified

(a) Description: Crystals

(b) Melting-point: 174-178°C

(c) Spectroscopy data: λ_{max} 257 nm in methanol; nuclear magnetic resonance and mass spectra are also given (Grasselli, 1973)

(d) Solubility: Soluble in water (0.1 g/100 ml), in ethanol (12.5 g/100 ml), in chloroform (2.5 g/100 ml), in ether (7.7 g/100 ml), in benzene (0.14 g/100 ml) and in alkaline hydroxides and carbonates

1.4 Technical products and impurities

Various national and international pharmacopoeias give specifications for the purity of phenobarbital in pharmaceutical products. For example, phenobarbital is available in the US as a USP grade containing 98-101% active ingredient on a dried basis. It is available in 7.5 and 20 mg doses per 5 ml of an elixir which contains 92.5-107.5% of the stated amount of phenobarbital. The alcoholic content of the elixir is 12 to 15% as ethanol. Phenobarbital tablets in doses of 8, 15, 25, 30, 60 and 100 mg are available containing 94-106% of the stated amount of phenobarbital. It is also available in powder form (US Pharmacopeial Convention, Inc., 1975). Combinations of 15 and 30 mg phenobarbital with 25 and 50 mg ephedrine sulphate in capsules, and of 8 mg phenobarbital with 130 mg theophylline and 24 mg ephedrine hydrochloride in tablet form are available (National Formulary Board, 1970). Phenobarbital is also formulated in a variety of combinations with other barbiturates and other drugs, such as scopolamine hydrobromide and phenyltoloxamine, for multiple medication therapy (Kastrup, 1976).

In Europe, phenobarbital preparations contain 99–101% active ingredient on a dried basis (Council of Europe, 1969). It is available in the UK in tablets, containing 92.5–107.5% active ingredient, and for injection (British Pharmacopoeia Commission, 1973).

In the USSR, phenobarbital is also available in tablets containing 20 mg phenobarbital, 250 mg theobromine and 20 mg papaverine hydrochloride (Mashkovski, 1972).

Phenobarbital sodium

1.1 Synonyms and trade names

Chem. Abstr. Reg. Serial No.: 57-30-7

Chem. Abstr. Name: 5-Ethyl-5-phenyl-2,4,6-(1H,3H,5H)pyrimidinetrione, monosodium salt

5-Ethyl-5-phenylbarbituric acid sodium; 5-ethyl-5-phenylbarbituric acid sodium salt; phenemalum; phenobarbital; phenobarbital elixir; phenobarbital-sodium; phenobarbitone sodium; phenobarbitone sodium salt; phenylethylbarbituric acid, sodium salt; sodium 5-ethyl-5-phenylbarbiturate; sodium phenobarbital; sodium phenobarbitone; sodium phenylethylbarbiturate; soluble phenobarbital; soluble phenobarbitone

Gardenal sodium; Luminal sodium; PBS; Phenobal sodium; Sodium luminal

1.2 Chemical formula and molecular weight

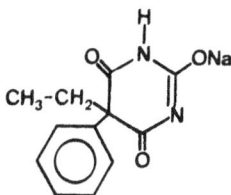

$C_{12}H_{11}N_2NaO_3$ Mol. wt: 254.2

159

1.3 Chemical and physical properties of the pure substance

From Stecher (1968)

(a) Description: Slightly hygroscopic crystals or white powder

(b) Solubility: Soluble in water (100 g/100 ml) and in ethanol
(10 g/100 ml); insoluble in ether and chloroform

(c) Stability: Aqueous solutions are stable for a few days at
10°C

1.4 Technical products and impurities

Various national and international pharmacopoeias give specifications
for the purity of phenobarbital sodium in pharmaceutical products. For
example, phenobarbital sodium is available in the US as a USP grade containing 98.5-101% active ingredient on a dried basis with a maximum of
0.003% heavy metals. Phenobarbital sodium injections are available in
doses of 60, 130 and 160 mg per ml as sterile solutions in a suitable
solvent (such as water, ethanol or propylene glycol) and contain 90-105%
of the stated amount. Sterile phenobarbital sodium suitable for parenteral
use is available in 60, 130, 200 and 320 mg doses. Tablets containing
35 mg phenobarbital sodium are also available. Phenobarbital sodium can
be obtained in powder form (US Pharmacopeial Convention, Inc., 1975).

In the UK, it is available on a dried basis containing no less than 98%
active ingredient and in tablets containing 92.5-107.5% of the stated
amount (British Pharmacopoeia Commission, 1973).

2. Production, Use, Occurrence and Analysis

For important background information on this section, see preamble,
p. 15.

2.1 Production and use

(a) Production

A method of preparing phenobarbital by ethylating phenylmalonic ester
followed by condensation with urea in the presence of sodium ethoxide was
first patented in Germany in 1911 (Stecher, 1968). Phenobarbital is

produced commercially in the following way: benzyl chloride is treated with sodium cyanide in methanol; the resulting benzyl cyanide is treated with a methanol-sulphuric acid mixture to yield methyl-phenylacetate; this is condensed with diethyl oxalate in sodium methoxide, and the resulting dimethyl-phenyloxalacetate is converted to dimethyl-phenylmalonate by heating *in vacuo*; this is ethylated with ethyl bromide in sodium methoxide, and the resulting ethylated ester is condensed with dicyanodiamide to give the iminobarbituric acid; this is hydrolysed with sulphuric acid, and crude phenobarbital is recrystallized from ethanol (Meyer & Rollet, 1964).

Phenobarbital sodium can be prepared by dissolving phenobarbital in an equivalent amount of sodium hydroxide solution in ethanol, followed by evaporation at low temperature (Swinyard, 1975).

Phenobarbital and phenobarbital sodium have been produced commercially in the US for over fifty years (US Tariff Commission, 1927). During the period 1950-1964, an average of 140,000 kg phenobarbital were produced annually in the US; in 1974, only two US companies reported production (see preamble, p. 15) (US International Trade Commission, 1976a). During the period 1955-1968, an average of 4700 kg phenobarbital sodium were produced annually in the US. In 1968, the last year in which separate US production data were reported, 5450 kg phenobarbital sodium were produced; only two US companies reported production (see preamble, p. 15) in 1974 (US International Trade Commission, 1976a). Current production of phenobarbital in the US is about 140,000 kg annually. US imports of phenobarbital through the principal customs districts were reported to be 14,400 kg in 1972 (US Tariff Commission, 1973), 500 kg in 1973 (US Tariff Commission, 1974) and the same amount in 1974 (US International Trade Commission, 1976b).

No evidence was found that phenobarbital or phenobarbital sodium is produced commercially in Japan; in 1975, less than 7,000 kg phenobarbital and less than 100 kg phenobarbital sodium were imported.

Annual production of phenobarbital in Europe is estimated to be in the range of 100-500 thousand kg: less than one thousand kg in Austria and in Benelux; and between 1-100 thousand kg in the Federal Republic of Germany, in France, in Hungary, in Italy, in Poland, in Scandinavia, in Spain, in Switzerland and in the UK.

Annual production of phenobarbital sodium in Europe is estimated to be in the range of 1-100 thousand kg: less than one thousand kg in Austria, in Benelux, in Scandinavia and in Spain; and 1-100 thousand kg in the Federal Republic of Germany, in France, in Hungary, in Italy, in Poland, in Switzerland and in the UK.

(b) Use

Phenobarbital and phenobarbital sodium are long-acting barbiturates used in human medicine as hypnotics, sedatives and in the treatment of epilepsy. When these compounds are used as hypnotics, they are administered orally in an average adult dose of 100 to 200 mg on retiring; the sodium salt may also be administered intravenously at a dose of 130-200 mg (Swinyard, 1975).

Phenobarbital or phenobarbital sodium can be used to produce mild, prolonged sedation for the treatment of conditions such as hypertension, functional gastrointestinal disorders, anxiety neuroses, coronary heart disease and preoperative apprehension. The average adult sedative dose is 15 to 30 mg orally two or three times daily; the sodium salt can be given by injection at a dose of 100-130 mg, repeated after 6 hours if necessary (Swinyard, 1975).

Phenobarbital and phenobarbital sodium are used in the treatment of epilepsy, especially for grand mal seizures, and are often employed in combination with a ketogenic diet, phenytoin or other therapeutic treatment. An average oral adult dose of either compound is 50 to 100 mg administered 2 or 3 times daily; the sodium salt can be administered parenterally in a dose of 200-320 mg, repeated after 6 hours if necessary (Swinyard, 1975).

Because of potential abuse leading to a limited physical or psycho-logical dependence, phenobarbital and phenobarbital sodium are classified in the US as controlled substances in Schedule IV of the Controlled Substances Act, which requires all manufacturers and distributors of these compounds to register and report to the US Drug Enforcement Agency any changes in the quantity manufactured or distributed and requires physicians to review their patients' status periodically (US Drug Enforcement Administration, 1976).

Total US sales of phenobarbital for use in human medicine are estimated to be less than 78,000 kg annually, and those of phenobarbital sodium, less than 2000 kg annually.

Phenobarbital is used in veterinary medicine as a sedative and anti-convulsant and in combination with dicyclomine hydrochloride to control nausea and vomiting (Siegmund, 1973). It is also reportedly used in the treatment of eclampsia, neuritis, pruritis, strychnine poisoning, as a preanaesthetic and as an anaesthetic (Stecher, 1968). Phenobarbital sodium is reportedly used in the same ways and, in addition, for the treatment of epileptiform convulsions (Stecher, 1968).

2.2 Occurrence

Neither phenobarbital nor phenobarbital sodium is known to occur in nature.

2.3 Analysis

A general review covers analytical methods for barbituric acid derivatives (Connors, 1961). Methods of assay for phenobarbital that meet regulatory requirements for pharmaceutical products include aqueous and non-aqueous titrations; those for phenobarbital sodium include gravimetry and spectrophotometry.

Spectrophotometric analysis has been used to determine phenobarbital in a mixture with caffeine and amidopyrine (Brutko & Sapegina, 1972). Phenobarbital sodium has been detected in mixtures containing bromides and a valerian tincture by UV spectrophotometry (Mosiniak, 1974). Another method, based on the combined use of UV spectrophotometry, volumetry and complexometry, can determine phenobarbital sodium in tablets containing ephedrine hydrochloride and calcium camphorsulphonate (Dobrecky, 1969).

Radioimmunoassays of phenobarbital have been reported (Cook *et al.*, 1975; Satoh *et al.*, 1974). Booker & Darcey (1975) made a comparison of enzymatic immunoassay and gas-liquid chromatography for the determination of phenobarbital. Polarographic methods can be used to determine pheno-barbital in barbiturate mixtures (Zuman, 1974) and in blood (Brooks *et al.*, 1973). Determination of phenobarbital, which has been separated from biological materials by fibre-glass instant thin-layer chromatography, has been accomplished by the use of a spectrophotofluorimetric method (Hsiung *et al.*, 1974).

For most gas chromatographic procedures phenobarbital is alkylated prior to its separation and determination. An extractive methylation technique is claimed to eliminate many of the complications associated with gas-chromatographic determinations (Ehrsson, 1974). More recent alkylation methods involve flash heating with the appropriate quaternary ammonium hydroxide (Friel & Troupin, 1975; Hooper *et al.*, 1975).

Quantitative thin-layer chromatographic methods have been developed for the determination of phenobarbital in the presence of other pharmaceutical compounds (Szasz & Dessouky, 1973) and for the determination of phenobarbital in biological fluids (Garceau *et al.*, 1973).

High-pressure liquid chromatographic methods are used to determine phenobarbital and phenytoin in biological materials (Atwell *et al.*, 1975; Evans, 1973) and phenobarbital in antispasmodic drug mixtures (Honigberg *et al.*, 1975).

A potentiometric titration assay for phenobarbital sodium uses perchloric acid as the titrant (Sell, 1968).

The methods of analysis used to determine phenobarbital in biological systems would, in principle, be applicable to phenobarbital sodium also.

3. Biological Data Relevant to the Evaluation of Carcinogenic Risk to Man

3.1 Carcinogenicity and related studies in animals

(a) Oral administration

Mouse: Phenobarbital sodium (purity not less than 98%) was administered for up to 109 weeks at a level of 500 mg per kg of diet to 30 male and 30 female 4-week old CF1 mice. When the experiment was terminated at 109 weeks, liver tumours were found in 24/30 males and 21/28 females, compared with 11/45 and 10/44, respectively, in the controls. The mortality rate in the treated group was no different from that of the controls, and tumour incidences at other sites were of the same order in both treated and control groups. Histologically, the liver tumours were classified as type A (in which parenchymal structure is basically retained) and type B (in which parenchymal structure is distorted). In the treated mice, there were 16 type A and 8 type B tumours in males and 12 type A and 9 type B tumours in females. In the controls there were 2 type B tumours in males, all other tumours being type A. No metastases were observed in this study; however, in a study reported in a footnote to the paper, the authors stated that when 1000 or 3000 mg phenobarbital sodium/kg of diet were administered in life-time tests, lung metastases were observed in mice with hepatocellular tumours of type B but not in those with type A (Thorpe & Walker, 1973).

The incidence of liver tumours in untreated 4 or 12-week old C3H mice (C3Hf/Anl)(Anl 70) caged in groups of five for 12 months was 7/17 in males and 1/16 in females. Addition of 500 mg phenobarbital/kg of diet raised these incidences to 16/17 and 10/16, respectively. In animals caged singly for 12 months, the incidences of hepatic tumours were 25/37 in males and 5/39 in females. The addition of 500 mg phenobarbital/kg of diet increased the incidence in animals caged singly to 35/36 and 29/29, respectively (Peraino et al., 1973a) [No evaluation of food intake was made in this study].

A group of 112 male and 74 female 4-week old CF1 mice received 0.05% phenobarbital sodium in the drinking-water for life (maximum duration, 120 weeks), and this group was compared with a group of 49 male and 47 female untreated controls. Survival at 80 weeks was about 50% in both groups and was reduced to about 5% in treated animals, compared with 15% in controls, at 120 weeks. The incidence of liver tumours in treated males was 77/98 and that in treated females 45/73, compared with 12/44 in male and 0/47 in female controls (the reference number is the effective number of mice surviving at the appearance of the first tumour). The incidences of other tumours were not increased in treated animals. Of the 122 parenchymal liver tumours observed in treated mice, 58 were classified as liver-cell carcinomas; no metastases were observed (Ponomarkov et al., 1976).

Rat: In a study in which the effect of phenobarbital on the incidence of acetylaminofluorene-induced liver carcinogenesis was observed, a control group of 48 3-week old male Sprague-Dawley rats were fed a diet containing 500 mg/kg of diet phenobarbital alone. No tumours were observed in this group within 64 weeks (Peraino et al., 1975) [The Working Group noted the short duration of this study].

Phenobarbital sodium was administered at a concentration of 500 mg/l in the drinking-water to 36 male and 34 female 7-week old Wistar rats for lifespan. Twenty-two males and 28 females were still alive when the first hepatic tumour appeared at about 99 weeks. At the termination of the experiment at 152 weeks of age, 13 males and 9 females had developed benign hepatic neoplasms. No hepatic tumours were observed in a comparable group of 36 male and 35 female control rats. The incidences of other neoplasms were comparable in test and control groups of rats (Rossi et al., 1976).

(b)   Intraperitoneal administration

Rat: A group of 36 male and 36 female 12-day old Sprague-Dawley rats received weekly i.p. injections of 2 mg/kg bw phenobarbital for life; mean survival times were 80 weeks in males and 85 weeks in females (significantly reduced in comparison with controls, in which they were 96 and 94 weeks, respectively). Among 32 males and 30 females surviving 200 or more days, 2 tumours were observed (a malignant tumour of the adrenal gland and 1 carcinoma of the nasal cavity). Among 36 male and 33 female controls, 1 haemangioendothelioma of the liver and 3 mammary adenocarcinomas were observed (Schmähl & Habs, 1976).

3.2   Other relevant biological data

(a)   Experimental systems

The i.p. LD_{50} of phenobarbital sodium in mice is 340 mg/kg (Collins & Horlington, 1969); the oral LD_{50} in rats is 660 mg/kg bw (Stecher, 1968).

After an i.v. injection to rats of 50 mg/kg bw ^{14}C-phenobarbital, the concentration in the liver is higher than that in other internal organs, and elimination in the urine reaches a peak after 6-8 hours (Glasson et al., 1959). Of a 75 mg/kg bw i.v. dose of phenobarbital sodium to male Sprague-Dawley rats, 18% was excreted in the bile in 6 hours as unidentified metabolites (Klaassen, 1971). Metabolites of phenobarbital sodium produced

166

in rats and guinea-pigs are 5-(3,4-dihydroxy-1,5-cyclohexadien-1-yl)-5-ethylbarbituric acid, 5-(1-hydroxyethyl)-5-phenylbarbituric acid, 5-(3,4-dihydroxyphenyl)-5-ethylbarbituric acid and 5-(4-hydroxyphenyl)-5-ethyl-barbituric acid (Harvey *et al*., 1972).

Since the observation that barbiturates stimulate drug metabolism (Remmer, 1958), several reviews have dealt with the extensively documented effect of phenobarbital on liver enlargement and with the induction of microsomal enzymes in various species, including man (Barka & Popper, 1967; Conney, 1967; Conney & Gelboin, 1972; Kunz *et al*., 1966; Mannering, 1971; Remmer, 1965; Schulte-Hermann, 1974). Phenobarbital-induced microsomal enzymes are characterized by a low substrate specificity. Consequently, they are involved in the metabolism of a large variety of endogenous and exogenous substances, e.g., in the activation and detoxification of chemical carcinogens. Therefore, phenobarbital treatment often leads to alterations in the biological activity of numerous compounds, including toxicity and carcinogenicity (Mitchell & Jollows, 1975; Wattenberg, 1975).

The simultaneous administration to rats of phenobarbital sodium with *N*-nitrosodiethylamine (NDEA), 2-acetylaminofluorene (AAF), 4-dimethylamino-azobenzene or aflatoxin reduced the production of hepatic tumours (Ishidate *et al*., 1967; Kunz *et al*., 1969; McLean & Marshall, 1971; Peraino *et al*., 1971; Takamiya *et al*., 1973; Weisburger *et al*., 1975). However, when phenobarbital was administered after treatment for a few weeks with AAF or NDEA, the hepatic tumour incidence was enhanced (Peraino *et al*., 1971, 1973b; Weisburger *et al*., 1975).

Phenobarbital administration does not alter the renal tumorigenic response to a single dose of *N*-nitrosodimethylamine in rats on a protein-free diet (McLean & Magee, 1970). It partially counteracted the carcinogenic effect of *N*-nitrosodibutylamine on the mouse bladder epithelium but failed to affect that of *N*-nitrosobutyl(4-hydroxybutyl)amine (Bertram & Craig, 1972).

The incidence of lung adenomas in mice after a single high dose of urethane was reduced when the mice were pretreated with several successive injections of phenobarbital (Adenis *et al*., 1970); but when the phenobarbital treatment was given after that of urethane, opposite results were obtained (De Azevedo e Silva, 1972).

No clear effects on skin carcinogenesis by polycyclic aromatic hydrocarbons were obtained, whether phenobarbital was administered simultaneously or some days or weeks after the carcinogens (Grube et al., 1975).

ICI pathogen-free mice were treated with phenobarbital sodium in the diet on days 6 to 16 of pregnancy: with 50 mg/kg of diet phenobarbital sodium, 0.6% of foetuses had cleft palates, and with 150 mg/kg, 3.9%, whereas there were very few cleft palates in untreated controls (0.3%) (Sullivan & McElhatton, 1975). An increased incidence of cleft palate was also reported in mice given s.c. injections of 175 mg/kg bw phenobarbital sodium between the 11th and 14th day after conception (Walker & Patterson, 1974).

Phenobarbital binds to rat chromatin *in vivo* (Alam & Steele, 1973). It has been reported to be weakly mutagenic in *Drosophila melanogaster* after addition of 2-3 mg (the LD_{50}) to the nutrient medium (Filippova et al., 1975); it did not induce point mutations in *Salmonella typhimurium* TA100, TA1535, TA1537 or TA98 (McCann & Ames, 1976; McCann et al., 1975).

(b) Man

Phenobarbital is readily absorbed from the gastrointestinal tract of man (Lous, 1954). Its metabolism seems to bear a close similarity to that reported in rats by Glasson & Benakis (1961). The major metabolite is the *para*-hydroxy derivative, which is excreted in the urine partly as the sulphate conjugate (Butler, 1956). For reviews of the action of phenobarbital as an enzyme inducer, see 3.2(a).

A possible association between maternal epilepsy, anticonvulsant drugs (mainly phenobarbital and phenytoin) and congenital malformations in offspring was reported by Meadow (1968). In two reports, a total of 38 children born to mothers who took anticonvulsants, including phenobarbital, throughout pregnancy revealed a similar constellation of malformations suggesting a syndrome involving lip and palate, cardiovascular system and skeletal abnormalities (limb, face, skull) (Meadow, 1968, 1970). Subsequent

case reports of epileptic women treated throughout pregnancy with phenobarbital and phenytoin have described affected infants with similar abnormalities (Aase, 1974; Anderson, 1976; Barr *et al.*, 1974; Dabee *et al.*,
1975; Loughnan *et al.*, 1973; Seip, 1976).

In 51 pregnancies identified from US hospital records over the period
1960-1970 occurring in 42 epileptic patients receiving phenobarbital and
phenytoin in 44 cases, and phenytoin alone or with mysoline in the other
cases, throughout pregnancy, 3 congenital abnormalities occurred (5.8%).
Although no anomalies were found in 50 matched pregnancies, the effect was
not considered to be statistically significant (Watson & Spellacy, 1971).

In the UK, 168 epileptic women treated with phenobarbital, phenytoin
or other anticonvulsant drugs were identified from the neurology departments of two general hospitals. These women had experienced 365 pregnancies,
during which phenobarbital alone or in combination was taken in 240 cases
and phenytoin alone, or in combination, in 192 cases. Seventeen of the
365 infants had malformations, compared with 7 of 483 controls and 0 of 62
offspring of epileptic women not taking medication. The calculated risk
was two to three times greater than normal (Speidel & Meadow, 1972).

During 1969 and 1970, 7,896 women gave birth at a single London
hospital, and 192 of the infants had malformations, to give a rate of
2.44%. In this group, 22 epileptic mothers had taken anticonvulsant drugs
throughout pregnancy. Two of the children born to mothers who had taken
phenobarbital and phenytoin in one case, and phenytoin and other drugs in
the other case, had cleft palate and/or hare lip, an incidence of 9%,
whereas only 0.13% of the infants born to non-epileptic mothers were so
affected (South, 1972).

In Cardiff, 31,877 infants born between 1965 and 1971 were studied;
245 mothers in this series had a history of epilepsy. Among the 111 births
to epileptic mothers not on anticonvulsant therapy, the malformation
rate was 2.7%, compared to 2.8% of infants in the total population. In
contrast, 6.7% of 134 infants born to mothers receiving anticonvulsant
therapy had malformations. One child had a hare lip but no cleft
palate among 53 born to mothers treated with phenobarbital alone; whereas

6 children were born with malformations among 60 births to mothers treated with phenobarbital and phenytoin (Lowe, 1973).

In a survey in Northern Ireland, the risk to infants born to epileptic mothers taking anticonvulsant drugs, mainly phenobarbital or phenytoin and other drugs, was 6.4% compared with a malformation rate of 3.8% for all live and stillbirths in the province. There was a 7-fold increase in the risk of cleft lip with or without cleft palate (1.8% compared with 0.22%) (Millar & Nevin, 1973).

In the Oxford Record Linkage Study, of live babies born between 1966 and 1970 to epileptic mothers, 17/217 (7.8%) had congenital abnormalities at birth compared with 21/649 (3.2%) of the controls matched for civil status, social class, maternal age, parity, hospital and year of delivery. Subsequently, the rates rose to 13.8% (30/217) for babies of epileptic mothers and 5.6% (36/649) for those in the control group [This may be due to a longer observation time and to the inclusion of different types of malformations, which may have been considered to be congenital before]. Maternal phenobarbital ingestion alone did not account for an increased incidence of defects (2/41, 4.9%) over that in infants of mothers not taking drugs (2/19, 10.5%), but when phenobarbital was given in combination with phenytoin the proportion of infants with defects was more than doubled (11/50, 22%). The incidence of defects among infants of mothers taking phenytoin alone (5/33, 15.2%), while higher than that among infants of mothers taking phenobarbital alone, was lower than that among infants of mothers taking phenytoin in combination with phenobarbital (Fedrick, 1973).

A study of pregnancies followed in a single US clinic included 284 births to 138 epileptic mothers between 1939 and 1972. Of 141 births to mothers taking anticonvulsants during the first trimester, 10 infants had malformations; of 56 births to epileptics not taking medication, 1 infant had a malformation; and of 26 births to epileptic mothers in remission no malformations were seen. The association of cleft palate and heart malformations with anticonvulsant usage was similar in 28 patients treated with phenobarbital alone and in 24 women treated with phenytoin alone (Annegers et al., 1974).

Barry & Danks (1974) reported that in Australia between 1967 and 1972, 10/39 infants born to mothers who were treated with phenytoin and barbiturates during pregnancy had congenital abnormalities. No congenital abnormalities were found in children of mothers treated with barbiturates alone, whereas they occurred in 2/8 children of those treated with phenytoin (see also monograph on phenytoin, p. 201).

After treatment with 22.4-388 µg/ml phenobarbital *in vitro*, a weak increase in the number of chromosome gaps and breaks was observed in cultivated peripheral human leucocytes (Foerst, 1972). No chromosome abnormalities were reported in human fibroblasts exposed *in vitro* to concentrations of 0.13-130 µg/ml for 5 days (Stenchever & Jarvis, 1970). Very high doses of phenobarbital (100-400 µg/ml) induced accumulation of metaphases in cultured human leucocytes; however, this study did not indicate if chromosome abnormalities were noted (Caratzali & Roman, 1969).

3.3 Case reports and epidemiological studies

(a) Case reports

Of 7 patients originally described by Saltzstein & Ackerman (1959) as developing pseudolymphomas following phenobarbital and/or phenytoin treatment, two died, one from multiple myeloma with an unknown survival time after diagnosis and another from malignant lymphoma, within 4 years (Harrington *et al.*, 1962).

Of 4 patients receiving phenobarbital and phenytoin, 2 were reported to have developed Hodgkin's disease, 1 a lymphosarcoma and 1 a reticulum-cell sarcoma (Hyman & Sommers, 1966) (see also monograph on phenytoin, p. 201).

Two cases of neuroblastoma, a 3-year old girl and a 7-day old boy, have been reported in the foetal hydantoin syndrome. Both mothers had taken anticonvulsants (phenobarbital and phenytoin) since girlhood because of epilepsy (Pendergrass & Hanson, 1976; Sherman & Roizen, 1976).

(b) Epidemiological studies

The carcinogenicity of anticonvulsant drugs, including phenobarbital, in man was studied in a retrospective investigation conducted on 9136 epileptic patients admitted to the neuropsychiatric hospital of Filadelfia in Denmark between 1933 and 1962. The patients were treated with pheno-barbital (100-300 mg), phenytoin (100-400 mg) or primidone (500-1500 mg). In those treated for up to 10 years, the incidence of cancer at all sites except the liver was the same as or lower than that expected when compared with the incidence in the general population. In patients treated for more than 10 years, 3 cases of liver cancer were observed in males whereas 1.1 were expected, and 1 liver cancer was observed in a female where 0.7 was expected; and in males treated for less than 10 years, 1 liver cancer was observed where 0.4 was expected. The author reported that one man with liver cancer had been treated with thorotrast 18 years before death. In patients treated for more than 10 years, tumours of brain and nervous system were observed in 10 males (expected 3.5) and in 6 females (expected 2.9) (see also 'General Remarks on Substances Considered', pp. 24-25) (Clemmesen *et al.*, 1974). Schneiderman (1974) reconsidered these results with respect to liver tumours and suggested that the cases of liver cancer might represent an increased incidence; but Clemmesen (1975) reported that 3 out of the 4 liver cancers seen in male patients had previously been treated with thorotrast, which is known to induce liver tumours in man (Kiely *et al.*, 1973; MacMahon *et al.*, 1947; Mann *et al.*, 1976; da Silva Horta *et al.*, 1965; Smoron & Bettifora, 1972).

4. Comments on Data Reported and Evaluation[1]

4.1 Animal data

Phenobarbital sodium is carcinogenic in mice and rats after its oral administration for lifetime. In mice, it produced benign and malignant liver-cell tumours; in rats, benign liver-cell tumours were observed very late in life.

---

[1]See also the section 'Animal Data in Relation to the Evaluation of Risk to Man' in the introduction to this volume, p. 13.

4.2 <u>Human data</u>

A possible relationship between anticonvulsant therapy in which phenobarbital was known to be included and the occurrence of cancer in man has been investigated in one large epidemiological study and reported in several case studies. In most instances, phenobarbital was given in conjunction with other drugs, in particular phenytoin. The available evidence is insufficient to allow an evaluation of the carcinogenicity of phenobarbital to be made (see also monograph on phenytoin, p. 201).

5. References

Aase, J.M. (1974) Anticonvulsant drugs and congenital abnormalities. Amer. J. Dis. Child., 127, 758

Adenis, L., Vlaeminck, M.N. & Driessens, J. (1970) L'adénome pulmonaire de la souris Swiss recevant de l'uréthane. VIII. Action du phéno-barbital. C.R. Soc. Biol. (Paris), 164, 560-562

Alam, S.N. & Steele, W.J. (1973) In vivo binding of phenobarbital (PB) and actinomycin D (AMD) to rat liver chromatin. Fed. Proc., 32, 684

Anderson, R.C. (1976) Cardiac defects in children of mothers receiving anticonvulsant therapy during pregnancy. J. Pediat., 89, 318-319

Annegers, J.F., Elveback, L.R., Hauser, W.A. & Kurland, L.T. (1974) Do anticonvulsants have a teratogenic effect? Arch. Neurol., 31, 364-373

Atwell, S.H., Green, V.A. & Haney, W.G. (1975) Development and evaluation of method for simultaneous determination of phenobarbital and diphenyl-hydantoin in plasma by high-pressure liquid chromatography. J. pharm. Sci., 64, 806-809

Barka, T. & Popper, H. (1967) Liver enlargement and drug toxicity. Medicine, 46, 103-117

Barr, M., Jr, Poznanski, A.K. & Schmickel, R.D. (1974) Digital hypoplasia and anticonvulsants during gestation : a teratogenic syndrome? J. Pediat., 84, 254-256

Barry, J.E. & Danks, D.M. (1974) Anticonvulsants and congenital abnormali-ties. Lancet, ii, 48-49

Bertram, J.S. & Craig, A.W. (1972) Specific induction of bladder cancer in mice by butyl-(4-hydroxybutyl)nitrosamine and the effects of hormonal modifications on the sex difference in response. Europ. J. Cancer, 8, 587-594

Booker, H.E. & Darcey, B.A. (1975) Enzymatic immunoassays vs. gas/liquid chromatography for determination of phenobarbital and diphenylhydantoin in serum. Clin. Chem., 21, 1766-1768

British Pharmacopoeia Commission (1973) British Pharmacopoeia, London, HMSO, pp. 358-359

Brooks, M.A., De Silva, J.A.F. & Hackman, M.R. (1973) Determination of phenobarbital and diphenylhydantoin in blood by differential pulse polarography. Analyt. chim. acta., 64, 165-175

Brutko, L.I. & Sapegina, L.P. (1972) Polybuffer-spectrophotometric analysis. Farmatsiya (Moscow), 21, 25-30

174

Butler, T.C. (1956) The metabolic hydroxylation of phenobarbital. J. Pharmacol. exp. Ther., 116, 326-336

Caratzali, A. & Roman, I.C. (1969) Action stathmocinétique de quelques dérivés barbituriques sur le lymphocyte human en culture. C.R. Acad. Sci. (Paris), Serie D, 268, 191-192

Clemmesen, J. (1975) Phenobarbitone, liver tumours and thorotrast. Lancet, i, 37-38

Clemmesen, J., Fuglsang-Frederiksen, V. & Plum, C.M. (1974) Are anti-convulsants oncogenic? Lancet, i, 705-707

Collins, A.J. & Horlington, M. (1969) A sequential screening test based on the running component of audiogenic seizures in mice, including reference compound PD50 values. Brit. J. Pharmacol., 37, 140-150

Conney, A.H. (1967) Pharmacological implications of microsomal enzyme induction. Pharmacol. Rev., 19, 317-366

Conney, A.H. & Gelboin, H.V. (1972) Drug-induced Diseases, 4, 179

Connors, K.A. (1961) Derivatives of carbamic acid. In: Higuchi, T. & Brockmann-Hanssen, E., eds, Pharmaceutical Analysis, New York, Interscience, pp. 181-263

Cook, C.E., Amerson, E., Poole, W.K., Lesser, P. & O'Tuama, L. (1975) Phenytoin and phenobarbital concentrations in saliva and plasma measured by radioimmunoassay. Clin. Pharmacol. Ther., 18, 742-747

Council of Europe (1969) European Pharmacopoeia, Vol. 1, 57-Sainte-Ruffine, France, Maisonneuve, pp. 346-348

Dabee, V., Hart, A.G. & Hurley, R.M. (1975) Teratogenic effects of diphenylhydantoin. Canad. med. Ass. J., 112, 75-76

De Azevedo e Silva, E. (1972) New data on the time-dependent inhibitory activity of post-treatment with phenobarbital on the lung carcinogenic action of ethyl urethane in white mice. Inst. Biocienc., Univ. Fed. Pernambuco, Recife, Brazil, Avulsa

Dobrecky, J. (1969) Quantitative determination of ephedrine hydrochloride, calcium camphorsulfonate, and sodium phenylethylbarbiturate in pharmaceutical compositions. Proanalisis, 2, 122-124

Ehrsson, H. (1974) Gas chromatographic determination of barbiturates after extractive methylation in carbon disulfide. Analyt. Chem., 46, 922-924

Evans, J.E. (1973) Simultaneous measurement of diphenylhydantoin and pheno-barbital in serum by high performance liquid chromatography. Analyt. Chem., 45, 2428-2429

Fedrick, J. (1973) Epilepsy and pregnancy: a report from the Oxford Record Linkage Study. Brit. med. J., ii, 442-448

Filippova, L.M., Rapoport, I.A., Shapiro, Y.L. & Alexandrovsky, Y.A. (1975) Mutagenic activity of psychotropic drugs. Genetika, 11, 77-82

Foerst, D. (1972) Chromosomenuntersuchungen nach der Einwirkung von Primidon (Mylepsinum[R]) und seiner Abbauprodukte Phenobarbital und Phenylethylmalondiamide in vitro. Acta genet. med. gemellol., 21, 305-318

Friel, P. & Troupin, A.S. (1975) Flash-heater ethylation of some anti-epileptic drugs. Clin. Chem., 21, 751-754

Garceau, Y., Philopoulos, Y. & Hasegawa, J. (1973) Quantitative TLC determination of primidone, phenylethylmalonediamide, and phenobarbital in biological fluids. J. pharm. Sci., 62, 2032-2034

Glasson, B. & Benakis, A. (1961) Etude du phénobarbital C-14 dans l'organisme du rat. Helv. physiol. acta, 19, 323-334

Glasson, B., Lerch, P. & Viret, J.-P. (1959) Etude du phénobarbital marqué dans l'organisme du rat. Helv. physiol. acta, 17, 146-152

Grasselli, J.G., ed. (1973) CRC Atlas of Spectral Data and Physical Constants for Organic Compounds, Cleveland, Ohio, Chemical Rubber Co., p. B-191

Grube, D.D., Peraino, C. & Fry, R.J.M. (1975) The effect of dietary phenobarbital on the induction of skin tumors in hairless mice with 7,12-dimethylbenz[a]anthracene. J. invest. Derm., 64, 258-262

Harrington, W.J., Tosteson, P.K., McAlister, W.H., Saltzstein, S.L., Brown, E., Restrepo, A., Fliedner, T.M., Loeb, V., Jr, Parker, B.M. & Kissane, Y. (1962) Lymphoma or drug reaction occurring during hydantoin therapy for epilepsy. Amer. J. Med., 32, 286-297

Harvey, D.J., Glazener, L., Stratton, C., Nowlin, J., Hill, R.M. & Horning, M.G. (1972) Detection of a 5-(3,4-dihydroxy-1,5-cyclo-hexadien-1-yl)-metabolite of phenobarbital and mephobarbital in rat, guinea pig and human. Res. Comm. chem. Path. Pharmacol., 3, 557-565

Honigberg, I.L., Stewart, J.T., Smith, A.P., Plunkett, R.D. & Justice, E.L. (1975) Liquid chromatography in pharmaceutical analysis. IV. Determination of antispasmodic mixtures. J. pharm. Sci., 64, 1389-1393

Hooper, W.D., Dubetz, D.K., Eadie, M.J. & Tyrer, J.H. (1975) Simultaneous assay of methylphenobarbitone and phenobarbitone using gas-liquid chromatography with on-column butylation. J. Chromat., 110, 206-209

Hsiung, M.W., Itiaba, K. & Crawhall, J.C. (1974) Spectrofluorometric method for the estimation of barbiturates separated by instant thin-layer chromatography. Clin. Biochem., 7, 45-51

Hyman, G.A. & Sommers, S.C. (1966) The development of Hodgkin's disease and lymphoma during anticonvulsant therapy. Blood, 28, 416-427

Ishidate, M., Watanabe, M. & Odashima, S. (1967) Effect of barbital on carcinogenic action and metabolism of 4-dimethylaminoazobenzene. Gann, 58, 267-281

Kastrup, E.K., ed. (1976) Facts and Comparisons, St Louis, Missouri, Facts and Comparisons, Inc., pp. 272b-273a; 277-280; 280a-280b; 282a-e; 283-283b

Kiely, J.M., Titus, J.L. & Orvis, A. (1973) Thorotrast-induced hepatoma presenting as hyperparathyroidism. Cancer, 31, 1312-1314

Klaassen, C.D. (1971) Biliary excretion of barbiturates. Brit. J. Pharmacol., 43, 161-166

Kunz, W., Schaude, G., Schmid, W. & Siess, M. (1966) Lebervergrösserung durch Fremdstoffe. Naunyn-Schmiedeberg's Arch. exp. Path. Pharmak., 254, 470-488

Kunz, W., Schaude, G. & Thomas, C. (1969) Die Beeinflussung der Nitrosamincarcinogenese durch Phenobarbital und Halogenkohlenwasserstoffe. Z. Krebsforsch., 72, 291-304

Loughnan, P.M., Gold, H. & Vance, J.C. (1973) Phenytoin teratogenicity in man. Lancet, i, 70-72

Lous, P. (1954) Plasma levels and urinary excretion of three barbituric acids after oral administration to man. Acta pharmacol. toxicol., 10, 147-165

Lowe, C.R. (1973) Congenital malformations among infants born to epileptic women. Lancet, ii, 9-10

MacMahon, H.E., Murphy, A.S. & Bates, M.I. (1947) Endothelial-cell sarcoma of liver following thorotrast injections. Amer. J. Path., 23, 585-611

Mann, N.S., Chaudhry, A., Thaler, S. & Sachder, A. (1976) Hepatoma induced by thorium dioxide. South. med. J., 69, 510-512

Mannering, G.J. (1971) Microsomal enzyme systems which catalyze drug metabolism. In: La Du, B.N., Mandel, H.G. & Way, E.L., eds, Fundamentals of Drug Metabolism and Drug Disposition, Baltimore, Williams & Wilkins, pp. 206-252

Mashkovski, M.D. (1972) Drug Compounds, Vol. 1, Moscow, Medizina, pp. 24-25

McCann, J. & Ames, B.N. (1976) Detection of carcinogens as mutagens in the *Salmonella*/microsome test: assay of 300 chemicals: discussion. Proc. nat. Acad. Sci. (Wash.), 73, 950-954

McCann, J., Choi, E., Yamasaki, E. & Ames, B.N. (1975) Detection of carcinogens as mutagens in the *Salmonella*/microsome test: assay of 300 chemicals. Proc. nat. Acad. Sci. (Wash.), 72, 5135-5139

McLean, A.E.M. & Magee, P.N. (1970) Increased renal carcinogenesis by dimethyl nitrosamine in protein deficient rats. Brit. J. exp. Path., 51, 587-590

McLean, A.E.M. & Marshall, A. (1971) Reduced carcinogenic effects of aflatoxin in rats given phenobarbitone. Brit. J. exp. Path., 52, 322-329

Meadow, S.R. (1968) Anticonvulsant drugs and congenital abnormalities. Lancet, ii, 1296

Meadow, S.R. (1970) Congenital abnormalities and anticonvulsant drugs. Proc. roy. Soc. Med., 63, 48-49

Meyer, R. & Rollet, M. (1964) Barbituric acid and barbiturates. In: Kirk, R.E. & Othmer, D.F., eds, Encyclopedia of Chemical Technology, 2nd ed., Vol. 3, New York, John Wiley and Sons, p. 67

Millar, J.H.D. & Nevin, N.C. (1973) Congenital malformations and anti-convulsant drugs. Lancet, i, 328

Mitchell, J.R. & Jollows, D.J. (1975) Metabolic activation of drugs to toxic substances. Gastroenterology, 68, 392-410

Mosiniak, T. (1974) Spectrometric determination of phenobarbital sodium in mixtures containing bromides and a valerian tincture. Farm. Pol., 30, 1111-1114

National Formulary Board (1970) National Formulary XIII, Washington DC, American Pharmaceutical Association, pp. 266-267, 695-696

Pendergrass, T.W. & Hanson, J.W. (1976) Fetal hydantoin syndrome and neuroblastoma. Lancet, ii, 150

Peraino, C., Fry, R.J.M. & Staffeldt, E. (1971) Reduction and enhancement by phenobarbital of hepatocarcinogenesis induced in the rat by 2-acetylaminofluorene. Cancer Res., 31, 1506-1512

Peraino, C., Fry, R.J.M. & Staffeldt, E. (1973a) Enhancement of spontaneous hepatic tumorigenesis in C3H mice by dietary phenobarbital. J. nat. Cancer Inst., 51, 1349-1350

Peraino, C., Fry, R.J.M., Staffeldt, E. & Kisieleski, W.E. (1973b) Effects of varying the exposure to phenobarbital on its enhancement of 2-acetylaminofluorene-induced hepatic tumorigenesis in the rat. Cancer Res., 33, 2701-2705

Peraino, C., Fry, R.J.M., Staffeldt, E. & Christopher, J.P. (1975)
    Comparative enhancing effects of phenobarbital, amobarbital, diphenyl-
    hydantoin, and dichlorodiphenyltrichloroethane on 2-acetylaminofluorene-
    induced hepatic tumorigenesis in the rat. Cancer Res., 35, 2884-2890

Ponomarkov, V., Tomatis, L. & Turusov, V. (1976) The effect of long-term
    administration of phenobarbitone in CF-1 mice. Cancer Lett., 1,
    165-172

Remmer, H. (1958) Die Beschleunigung des Evipanabbaues unter der Wirkung
    von Barbituraten. Naturwissenschaften, 45, 189

Remmer, H. (1965) The fate of drugs in the organism. Ann. Rev. Pharmacol.,
    5, 405-428

Rossi, L., Ravera, M., Repetti, G. & Santi, L. (1976) The effect of long-
    term administration of DDT or phenobarbital-Na in Wistar rats.
    Int. J. Cancer (in press)

Saltzstein, S.L. & Ackerman, L.V. (1959) Lymphadenopathy induced by anti-
    convulsant drugs and mimicking clinically and pathologically malignant
    lymphomas. Cancer, 12, 164-182

Satoh, H., Kuroiwa, Y., Hamada, A. & Uematsu, T. (1974) Radioimmunoassay
    for phenobarbital. J. Biochem. (Tokyo), 75, 1301-1306

Schmähl, D. & Habs, M. (1976) Life-span investigations for carcinogenicity
    of some immune-stimulating, immunodepressive and neurotropic substances
    in Sprague-Dawley rats. Z. Krebsforsch., 86, 77-84

Schneiderman, M.A. (1974) Phenobarbitone and liver tumours. Lancet, ii,
    1085

Schulte-Hermann, R. (1974) Induction of liver growth by xenobiotic
    compounds and other stimuli. CRC Crit. Rev. Toxicol., September, 97-158

Seip, M. (1976) Growth retardation, dysmorphic facies and minor malfor-
    mations following massive exposure to phenobarbitone in utero.
    Acta paediat. scand., 65, 617-621

Sell, E. (1968) Potentiometric titration of certain basic compounds and
    their mixtures in differentiating solvents. Acta pol. pharm., 25,
    569-575

Sherman, S. & Roizen, N. (1976) Fetal hydantoin syndrome and neuroblastoma.
    Lancet, ii, 517

Siegmund, O.H., ed. (1973) The Merck Veterinary Manual, 4th ed., Rahway,
    NJ, Merck & Co., pp. 1525 and 1535

da Silva Horta, J., Abbatt, J.D., da Motta, L.C. & Roriz, M.L. (1965) Malignancy and other late effects following administration of thorotrast. Lancet, ii, 201-205

Smoron, G.L. & Battifora, H.A. (1972) Thorotrast-induced hepatoma. Cancer, 30, 1252-1259

South, J. (1972) Teratogenic effect of anticonvulsants. Lancet, ii, 1154

Speidel, B.D. & Meadow, S.R. (1972) Maternal epilepsy and abnormalities of the fetus and newborn. Lancet, ii, 839-843

Stecher, P.G., ed. (1968) The Merck Index, 8th ed., Rahway, NJ, Merck & Co., pp. 119 and 809

Stenchever, M.A. & Jarvis, J.A. (1970) Effect of barbiturates on the chromosomes of human cells in vitro - a negative report. J. reprod. Med., 5, 69-71

Sullivan, F.M. & McElhatton, P.R. (1975) Teratogenic activity of the anti-epileptic drugs phenobarbital, phenytoin and primidone in mice. Toxicol. appl. Pharmacol., 34, 271-282

Swinyard, E.A. (1975) Sedatives and hypnotics. In: Osol, A. et al., eds, Remington's Pharmaceutical Sciences, 15th ed., Easton, Pa, Mack, p. 1002

Szasz, G. & Dessouky, Y.M. (1973) Thin-layer chromatographic (TLC) separation and identification of barbiturates. Quantitative determination of phenobarbitone in the presence of other pharmaceutical compounds. Egypt. J. pharm. Sci., 14, 223-235

Takamiya, K., Chen, S-H. & Kitagawa, H. (1973) Effect of phenobarbital and DL-ethionine on 4-(dimethylamino)azobenzene-metabolizing enzymes and carcinogenesis. Gann, 64, 363-372

Thorpe, E. & Walker, A.I.T. (1973) The toxicology of dieldrin (HEOD). II. Comparative long-term oral toxicity studies in mice with dieldrin, DDT, phenobarbitone, β-BHC and γ-BHC. Fd Cosmet. Toxicol., 11, 433-442

US Drug Enforcement Administration (1976) Schedules of controlled substances. US Code of Federal Regulations, Title 21, part 1308.14, p. 76

US International Trade Commission (1976a) Synthetic Organic Chemicals, US Production and Sales, 1974, USITC Publication 776, Washington DC, US Government Printing Office, p. 105

US International Trade Commission (1976b) Imports of Benzenoid Chemicals and Products, 1974, USITC Publication 762, Washington DC, US Government Printing Office, p. 85

US Pharmacopeial Convention, Inc. (1975) The US Pharmacopeia, 19th rev., Rockville, Md, pp. 372-375

US Tariff Commission (1927) Census of Dyes and other Synthetic Organic Chemicals, 1926, Tariff Information Series No. 35, Washington DC, US Government Printing Office, p. 70

US Tariff Commission (1973) Imports of Benzenoid Chemicals and Products, 1972, TC Publication 601, Washington DC, US Government Printing Office, p. 83

US Tariff Commission (1974) Imports of Benzenoid Chemicals and Products, 1973, TC Publication 688, Washington DC, US Government Printing Office, p. 79

Walker, B.E. & Patterson, A. (1974) Induction of cleft palate in mice by tranquilizers and barbiturates. Teratology, 10, 159-164

Watson, J.D. & Spellacy, W.N. (1971) Neonatal effects of maternal treatment with the anticonvulsant drug diphenylhydantoin. Obstet. Gynec., 37, 881-885

Wattenberg, L.W. (1975) Effects of dietary constituents on the metabolism of chemical carcinogens. Cancer Res., 35, 3326-3331

Weisburger, J.H., Madison, R.M., Ward, J.M., Viguera, C. & Weisburger, E.K. (1975) Modification of diethylnitrosamine liver carcinogenesis with phenobarbital but not with immunosuppression. J. nat. Cancer Inst., 54, 1185-1188

Zuman, P. (1974) Polarography in the study of some analytically important reactions. Proc. Soc. analyt. Chem., 11, 338-340

PHENYLBUTAZONE AND OXYPHENBUTAZONE

1. Chemical and Physical Data

Phenylbutazone

1.1 Synonyms and trade names

Chem. Abstr. Reg. Serial No.: 50-33-9

Chem. Abstr. Name: 4-Butyl-1,2-diphenyl-3,5-pyrazolidinedione

4-Butyl-1,2-diphenyl-3,5-dioxopyrazolidine; 4-butyl-1,2-diphenyl-pyrazolidine-3,5-dione; 3,5-dioxo-1,2-diphenyl-4-n-butylpyrazo-lidine; diphebuzol; diphenylbutazone; 1,2-diphenyl-4-butyl-3,5-pyrazolidinedione; 1,2-diphenyl-3,5-dioxo-4-butylpyrazolidine; 1,2-diphenyl-3,5-dioxo-4-n-butylpyrazolidine; 1,2-diphenyl-2,3-dioxo-4-n-butylpyrazolidine; fenibutazona; fenylbutazon

Alindor; Alkabutazona; Alqoverin; Anerval; Anpuzone; Antadol; Anuspiramin; Arthrizin; Artrizin; Artrizone; Artropan; Azdid; Azobutil; Benzone; Betazed; Bizolin 200; B.T.Z.; Butacote; Butacompren; Butadion; Butadiona; Butadione; Butagesic; Butalgina; Butalan; Butalidon; Butaluy; Butaphen; Buta-Phen; Butapirazol; Butapyrazole; Butarecbon; Butartril; Butartrina; Butazina; Butazolidin; Butazolidine; Butazona; Butazone; Butidiona; Butiwas-simple; Butone; Butoz; Butylpyrin; Buvetzone; Buzon; Chembutazone; Digibutina; Diossidone; Diozol; Diphebuzol; Ecobutazone; Elmedal; Equi Bute; Eributazone; 'Esteve'; Febuzina; Fenartil; Fenibutasan; Fenibutol; Fenilbutazona; Fenilbutina; Fenilbutine; Fenilidina; Fenotone; Flexazone; G 13,871; IA-But; Intalbut; Intrabutazone; Ipsoflame; Kadol; Lingel; Malgesic; Mephabutazone; Merizone; Nadazone; Nadozone; Neo-Zoline; Novophenyl; Phebuzin; Phebuzine; Phen-Buta-Vet; Phenbutazol; Phenopyrine; Phenylbetazone; Phenylbutaz; Phenylbutazonum; Phenyl-Mobuzon; Pirarreumol 'B'; Praecirheumin; Pyrabutol; Pyrazolidin; Rectofasa; Reudo; Reudox; Reumasyl; Reumazin; Reumazol; Reumune; Reupolar; Robizon-V; Rubatone; Scanbutazone; Schemergin; Shigrodin; Tazone; Tetnor; Tevcodyne; Therazone; Ticinil; Todalgil; Uzone; VAC-10; Wescozone; Zolaphen; Zolidinum

1.2 Chemical formula and molecular weight

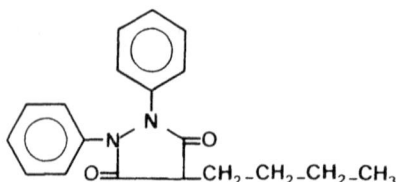

$$C_{19}H_{20}N_2O_2 \qquad \text{Mol. wt: } 308.4$$

1.3 Chemical and physical properties of the pure substance

From Stecher (1968), unless otherwise specified

(a) Description: Crystals

(b) Melting-point: $105^{\circ}C$

(c) Spectroscopy data: λ_{max} 239.5 nm ($E_1^1 = 516.2$) in acidic methanol; 264 nm in sodium hydroxide solution (US Pharmacopeial Convention, Inc., 1975)

(d) Solubility: Soluble in water, 70 mg/100 ml at $22.5^{\circ}C$ (also reported as 220 mg/100 ml)

1.4 Technical products and impurities

Various national and international pharmacopoeias give specifications for the purity of phenylbutazone in pharmaceutical products. For example, phenylbutazone is available in the US as a USP grade containing 98-100.5% active ingredient on a dried basis with a maximum of 0.001% heavy metals. Tablets are available in 100 mg doses containing 93-107% of the stated amount of phenylbutazone (US Pharmacopeial Convention, Inc., 1975). Capsules are also available in which 100 mg phenylbutazone (or 50 mg phenylbutazone and 1.25 mg prednisone) is combined with 100 mg dried aluminium hydroxide gel and 150 mg magnesium trisilicate (antacids added to minimize gastric upset) (Kastrup, 1976).

In the UK, phenylbutazone is available as suppositories (250 mg) containing 92.5-107.5% of the stated amount and as tablets (100 mg) containing 95-105% of the stated amount (British Pharmacopoeia Commission, 1973).

Oxyphenbutazone

1.1 Synonyms and trade names

Chem. Abstr. Reg. Serial No.: 129-20-4

Chem. Abstr. Name: 4-Butyl-1-(4-hydroxyphenyl)-2-phenyl-3,5-pyrazolidinedione

4-Butyl-2-(4-hydroxyphenyl)-1-phenyl-3,5-dioxopyrazolidine; 4-butyl-1-(*para*-hydroxyphenyl)-2-phenyl-3,5-pyrazolidinedione; 4-butyl-2-(*para*-hydroxyphenyl)-1-phenyl-3,5-pyrazolidinedione; hydroxyphenyl-butazone; *para*-hydroxyphenylbutazone; 1-(*para*-hydroxyphenyl)-2-phenyl-4-butyl-3,5-pyrazolidinedione; 1-*para*-hydroxyphenyl-2-phenyl-3,5-dioxo-4-*n*-butylpyrazolidine; metabolite I; oxazolidin; oxiphen-butazone; oxyphenobutazone; oxyphenylbutazone; *para*-oxyphenylbuta-zone; 1-phenyl-2-(*para*-hydroxyphenyl)-3,5-dioxo-4-butylpyrazolidine; 1-phenyl-2-(*para*-hydroxyphenyl)-3,5-dioxo-4-*n*-butylpyrazolidine

Artroflog; Butaflogin; Butanova; Butapirone; Butilene; Crovaril; Deflogin; Etrozolidina; Flamaril; Flanaril; Flogal; Floghene; Flogistin; Flogitolo; Flogodin; Flogoril; Flogostop; Flogirina; Frabel; G 27202; Idrobutazina; Infamil; Inflammil; Ipabutona; Iridil; Isobutazina; Isobutil; Neo-Farmadol; Neofen; Offitril; Oxalid; Oxazolidin-Geigy; Oxibutol; Oxi-Fenibutol; Pirabutina; Piraflogin; Poliflogil; Remazin; Reumox; Rumapax; Tandacote; Tandalgesic; Tandearil; Tanderal; Tanderil; Telidal; Tendearil; Validil; Visubutina

1.2 Chemical formula and molecular weight

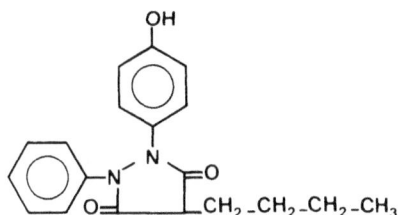

$C_{19}H_{20}N_2O_3$ Mol. wt: 324.4

1.3 Chemical and physical properties of the pure substance

From Stecher (1968), unless otherwise specified

(a) <u>Description</u>: Crystals

(b) <u>Melting-point</u>: 124-125°C

(c) <u>Spectroscopy data</u>: λ_{max} 254 nm in sodium hydroxide solution (National Formulary Board, 1970)

(d) <u>Solubility</u>: Soluble in benzene, chloroform, ethanol, ether and methanol

1.4 Technical products and impurities

Various national and international pharmacopoeias give specifications for the purity of oxyphenbutazone in pharmaceutical products. For example, oxyphenbutazone is available in the US as a National Formulary grade containing 98-100.5% active ingredient on an anhydrous basis. Tablets are available in 100 mg doses which contain 94-106% of the stated amount of oxyphenbutazone (National Formulary Board, 1970).

In the UK, oxyphenbutazone is available on a dried basis containing no less than 99% of the active ingredient and as tablets (dose 100 mg) containing 95-105% of the stated amount (British Pharmacopoeia Commission, 1973).

2. Production, Use, Occurrence and Analysis

For important background information on this section, see preamble, p. 15.

2.1 Production and use

(a) Production

A method of preparing phenylbutazone was patented in the US in 1951, in which butylmalonyl chloride is condensed with hydrazobenzene in ether solution with pyridine. Aqueous hydrochloric acid is used to extract the pyridine, and phenylbutazone is extracted with aqueous sodium carbonate. The alkaline solution is acidified with hydrochloric acid to give phenylbutazone (Stenzl, 1951).

A method of preparing oxyphenbutazone was patented in the US in 1956 and involves the following steps: diethyl butylmalonate is condensed with *para*-benzyloxyhydrazobenzene in a solution of sodium ethoxide in anhydrous ether; the addition of xylene forms 1-(*para*-benzyloxy)-2-phenyl-4-butyl-3,5-pyrazolidinedione; this is debenzylated by Raney nickel hydrogenation to give oxyphenbutazone (Häfliger, 1956).

Commercial production of phenylbutazone was first reported in the US in 1965 (US Tariff Commission, 1967); only one US company reported production (see preamble, p. 15) in 1974 (US International Trade Commission, 1976a). US imports of phenylbutazone through the principal customs districts were 2700 kg in 1972 (US Tariff Commission, 1973), 15,300 kg in 1973 (US Tariff Commission, 1974) and 10,300 kg in 1974 (US International Trade Commission, 1976b).

Commercial production of oxyphenbutazone was first reported in the US in 1960 (US Tariff Commission, 1961); only one US company reported production (see preamble, p. 15) in 1974 (US International Trade Commission, 1976a). US imports of oxyphenbutazone through the principal customs districts were 10 kg in 1972 (US Tariff Commission, 1973) and 175 kg in 1973 (US Tariff Commission, 1974).

Production of phenylbutazone was first reported in Japan in 1957; 1 major company and 10 smaller firms manufactured phenylbutazone in 1975. Over 50,000 kg phenylbutazone were used in Japan during that year. No evidence was found that oxyphenbutazone has ever been produced commercially in Japan; about 800 kg were imported in 1975.

Production of phenylbutazone in India in 1972 was reported to be at least 8900 kg. Imports for the period 1972-1973 were reported to be 24,180 kg (Anon., 1974).

Estimated annual production of phenylbutazone in Europe is estimated to be in the range of 100-500 thousand kg. Annual production is believed to be less than 1 thousand kg in Austria and in Benelux, and 1-100 thousand kg in the Federal Republic of Germany, in France, in Hungary, in Italy, in Poland, in Scandinavia, in Switzerland and in the UK. Annual production of oxyphenbutazone in Italy and in Spain is estimated to be in the range of

1-100 thousand kg; Scandinavia produces about 200 kg oxyphenbutazone annually for captive use only as a chemical intermediate.

(b) Use

Phenylbutazone and oxyphenbutazone are anti-inflammatory agents possessing analgesic, antipyretic, sodium retention and mild uricosuric properties (American Society of Hospital Pharmacists, 1961).

Both compounds are used in the symptomatic treatment of acute gout and to relieve the symptoms of rheumatoid arthritis, rheumatoid spondylitis, osteoarthritis and psoriatic arthritis; they are used in the symptomatic treatment of acute superficial thrombophlebitis and for severe forms of a variety of acute local inflammatory conditions (Kastrup, 1976).

When phenylbutazone is used to treat gout, a disease which afflicts about 800,000 people in the US (Cavallito, 1968), an initial oral dosage of 600 to 800 mg is administered on the first day of an acute attack, and the dose is reduced as the inflammation subsides (Knott, 1974).

Total US sales of phenylbutazone for use in human medicine are estimated to be less than 35,000 kg annually; those of oxyphenbutazone are less than 10,000 kg annually.

Phenylbutazone is also used in veterinary medicine as an analgesic, antipyretic and anti-inflammatory agent (Stecher, 1968).

2.2 Occurrence

Phenylbutazone and oxyphenbutazone are not known to occur in nature.

2.3 Analysis

Methods of assay for phenylbutazone that meet regulatory requirements for pharmaceutical products include aqueous and non-aqueous titration and spectrophotometry; those for oxyphenbutazone include aqueous titration and UV spectrophotometry.

Spectrophotometric methods developed for the assay of phenylbutazone (Magalhaes & Piros, 1973) include one based on the detection of the permanganate oxidation product of phenylbutazone following its extraction from plasma (Jähnchen & Levy, 1972).

188

Phenylbutazone can be analysed in plasma by high-speed liquid chromatography (Pound *et al.*, 1974), and levels of 0.25 µg/ml oxyphenbutazone can be determined in plasma by this method (Pound & Sears, 1975).

Gas-liquid chromatographic methods for determining phenylbutazone and oxyphenbutazone as their silyl derivatives in plasma have been described (Midha *et al.*, 1974; Tanimura *et al.*, 1975). Comparisons have been made of a gas chromatographic method and a UV-spectrophotometric method for the determination of phenylbutazone (McGilveray *et al.*, 1974) and of oxyphenbutazone in biological fluids (Bruce *et al.*, 1974). A gas chromatographic method for the determination of bulk and dosage forms of phenylbutazone has been reported (Watson *et al.*, 1973).

Phenylbutazone can also be analysed by thin-layer chromatographic methods (Krechniak *et al.*, 1972; Pomazánska-Kołodziejska, 1972; Saršúnová & Kakáč, 1972) or electrochemically by voltammetry (Proksa *et al.*, 1974) or alternating-current oscillopolarography (Szyszko & Weglowska, 1974).

3. Biological Data Relevant to the Evaluation of Carcinogenic Risk to Man

3.1 Carcinogenicity and related studies in animals

No data were available to the Working Group.

3.2 Other relevant biological data

(a) Experimental systems

The oral LD_{50} of phenylbutazone in mice is 680 mg/kg bw, that in rats 1000 mg/kg bw and that in rabbits 146 mg/kg bw; the i.v. LD_{50} in mice is 120 mg/kg bw and that in rats 150 mg/kg bw. The oral LD_{50} of oxyphenbutazone in dogs is 575 mg/kg bw; the i.v. LD_{50} in rats is 105 mg/kg bw (Sunshine, 1969).

Gastric ulcerations were produced in dogs after prolonged i.m. administration of doses of 3.6-35.2 g phenylbutazone over 10-103 days (Kirsner & Ford, 1955).

The biological half-life of phenylbutazone in plasma was about 6 hours in dogs, 5 hours in guinea-pigs and 3 hours in rabbits (Burns *et al.*, 1953).

Negative results have been reported with phenylbutazone in *Salmonella typhimurium* TA100, TA98, TA1535 and TA1537 in the presence or absence of rat liver homogenate (McCann & Ames, 1976; McCann *et al.*, 1975). It did not induce non-disjunction or crossing-over in *Aspergillus nidulans* in the absence of metabolic activation, whereas its metabolite, oxyphenbutazone, had weak but significant activity (Bignami *et al.*, 1974). Negative results were also obtained with phenylbutazone in the dominant lethal test following administration of the drug either to male mice at 50-100 mg/kg bw by i.p. injection (Machemer & Hess, 1971) or to female mice as a single oral dose of 400 mg/kg bw (Machemer & Hess, 1973).

No increase in the number of chromosome abnormalities has been observed in bone-marrow cells of Chinese hamsters after oral administration (Müller & Strasser, 1971) or of rats after i.p. administration of phenylbutazone (Gebhart & Wissmüller, 1973) or in germinal cells of male mice after oral administration (Rathenberg & Müller, 1972).

(b) Man

Administration of phenylbutazone to man is associated with peptic ulcer, hypersensitivity reactions, hepatitis, nephritis and bone-marrow suppression. The toxicity of oxyphenbutazone is similar to that of the parent compound (Mauer, 1955; Woodbury & Fingl, 1975).

The biological half-life of phenylbutazone in plasma is 72 hours (Burns *et al.*, 1953). Phenylbutazone given at 2-3 times the therapeutic dose is metabolized slowly, with the accumulation of oxyphenbutazone in the plasma. Oxyphenbutazone and γ-hydroxyphenylbutazone were excreted in the urine; no glucuronic acid conjugates of phenylbutazone were detected. In man, oxyphenbutazone has a biological half-life of about 2 days (Burns *et al.*, 1955).

Significant increases in the number of chromosome abnormalities resulting from chromosome breakage events were reported in cultured human peripheral leucocytes from patients treated with phenylbutazone for rheumatic disorders for at least 3 months in doses ranging from 100-500 mg/day. In the same study, a few of the patients were examined for chromosome damage in bone-marrow cells, with negative results (Stevenson *et al.*, 1971).

Negative results have also been reported for chromosome damage in bone-marrow cells from humans receiving 400 mg/day phenylbutazone for 1 week (Jensen, 1972). *In vitro* treatment of human leucocytes with 0.62-2.16 x 10^{-3} M/1 phenylbutazone caused an increased incidence of chromosome abnormalities (Wissmüller, 1971; Wissmüller & Gebhart, 1970).

3.3 Case reports and epidemiological studies

(a) Case reports

Six cases of leukaemia in patients who had received phenylbutazone were reported by Bean (1960). In case 1, a male aged 69 years was treated with 600 mg then 400 mg phenylbutazone daily for 3 weeks, when he developed a mild anaemia, leucocytosis and lymphadenopathy in the neck and axillae. He died 20 months after the beginning of treatment and *post mortem* showed myeloid leukaemia. Case 2 was a male aged 67 years who had suffered from lumbar spondylitis for many years and who had been treated with phenyl-butazone intermittently over 4 years prior to a terminal lymphatic leukaemia. Case 3 was a male aged 70 years who had been treated with 200-600 mg phenyl-butazone, then with an increased dose daily for 5 months prior to admission to hospital. Investigations revealed that he was suffering from lymphatic leukaemia, and he died 3 weeks later. In case 4, the period of treatment with phenylbutazone was approximately 1 year before death from myeloid leukaemia. The patient was a male aged 80 years and had suffered from osteoarthritis and spondylitis for many years. There was a history of some intolerance to phenylbutazone. Case 5, a male aged 66 years, had been treated with 600 then 100 mg/day phenylbutazone for 4 years before admission to hospital for acute diarrhoea and had tolerated the drug well. During investigation it was found that he had generalized lymphadenopathy and splenomegaly. Histological examination of the lymph nodes revealed the presence of malignant lymphoproliferative disease. Case 6, a 63-year old male, had received a course of fifty 100-mg phenylbutazone tablets approxi-mately 18 months before admission to hospital for severe angina. Three weeks after admission his blood picture was suggestive of myeloid leukaemia, confirmed at necropsy six days later.

Lawrence (1960) reported a leukaemoid reaction in a woman aged 69 1 month after treatment with 8.4 g phenylbutazone spread over 4 weeks, while

Garrett (1961) reported a similar reaction in a 64-year old woman who had taken 18 g phenylbutazone spread over 3 months. The blood dyscrasia was discovered a few weeks after cessation of treatment.

Cast (1961) mentioned some degree of intolerance to phenylbutazone in a female aged 59 after the administration of 300 mg daily for two months. Drug therapy was resumed after a respite of 14 months, when she was admitted for an operative procedure for the relief of osteoarthritis. During routine blood investigations, myeloid leukaemia was diagnosed and she died 14 days after operation.

Cadman & Limont (1962) reported a case of acute leukaemia in a 71-year old man who 3 months earlier had been treated with 20 200 mg phenylbutazone tablets over 6 days.

Chatterjea (1964) drew attention to a case of acute myeloid leukaemia in a 46-year old male who had taken phenylbutazone intermittently for a significant period prior to the onset of leukaemia.

A 56-year old female was treated with 300 mg phenylbutazone daily for 17 days. After 2 weeks she became seriously ill and was found to have an aplastic anaemia which was accompanied by extensive bruising; she died a week later. Autopsy showed massive cerebral haemorrhage, and diagnosis was of an acute leukaemia (Thorpe, 1964).

Chalmers & McCarthy (1964) described the onset of a fatal myelomono-cytic leukaemia in a 44-year old women treated with daily doses of 100-300 mg phenylbutazone for consecutive periods of 12, 8 and 19 months for rheumatoid arthritis.

Hart (1964) reported on a 58-year old man who was treated with 400 mg phenylbutazone daily for 7 days on two occasions separated by an interval of approximately 16 months. Two weeks after the second episode he developed acute myeloid leukaemia.

Golding et al. (1965) reported a case of fatal monocytic leukaemia after treatment for crippling rheumatoid arthritis with phenylbutazone in doses of 300 mg daily for one year and thereafter at 200 mg daily for about 4 years more. The patient's sister had died of the same disease at the age of 61 without ever having received phenylbutazone.

Five cases of acute leukaemia following phenylbutazone therapy, from a total of 55 cases of acute leukaemia observed in Australia in the years 1959-1963 were reported by Woodliff & Dougan (1964); 3 further cases associated with phenylbutazone treatment were reported by Dougan & Woodliff (1965). Of the total of 8 cases, 5 were in men and 3 in women; the doses ranged from approximately 3-100 g and the duration of treatment lasted from 1 week to 4 years continuously, or 7 years intermittently. The first symptoms related to leukaemia were observed from a few weeks to 1 year after cessation of phenylbutazone administration. Four other cases were excluded because of short duration of treatment or prior radiotherapy. Dougan & Woodliff (1965) also reported 4 cases of chronic myleoproliferative disorders (2 of Hodgkin's disease, 1 chronic lymphatic leukaemia and 1 polycythaemia vera) following administration of phenylbutazone for periods ranging from a few weeks to 2 years. The doses in two of these cases were about 6 and 45 g; in the other two they were unknown.

Three cases of acute leukaemia following phenylbutazone therapy, out of 50 cases of acute leukaemia, were recorded in Scandinavia between 1959 and 1964 (Jensen & Roll, 1965). A 78-year old male was given 600 mg phenylbutazone daily for 4 months. In the following month he was admitted to hospital with anaemia, and haematological investigations revealed the early stages of myelocytic leukaemia, from which the patient died approximately 13 months later. The second case concerned a 67-year old man who received 300 mg daily for a few months for rheumatoid arthritis. Shortly afterwards he had an acute episode of gastrointestinal haemorrhage from which he recovered, but 2 years later he died of acute myeloblastic leukaemia. The third case was a comparatively young female, 31 years of age, given repeated courses of phenylbutazone in doses of 400-600 mg daily for 10 days. About 14 months later she was admitted to hospital with severe anaemia, and a haematological investigation revealed lymphoblastic leukaemia; she died one year later.

Acute leukaemia, or a leukaemoid reaction, has also been observed after treatment with oxyphenbutazone. In one case, a 30-year old woman suffering from mild myasthenia gravis was given approximately 5 g oxyphenbutazone over a month. Shortly afterwards, she developed an anaemia, a leucocytosis; this was followed by leucocytopenia, which became steadily worse over a period of 26 days of observation but showed signs of improvement after 11 months. In a second case, a 40-year old man received a total dose of 1 g oxyphenbutazone over approximately 5 days, 2 months before admission to hospital with a severe anaemia and leucocytosis; he died on the third day after developing this condition. The third case concerned a 32-year old woman who was treated with 2.5 g oxyphenbutazone over 7 days; she also developed severe leucocytosis followed by leucopenia and anaemia, but there was a subsequent recovery. The last case of white-blood cell disorder concerned a 47-year old man who, 13 months before admission with a temperature, had been given 1.9 g oxyphenbutazone over a 2-week period. On admission, he was given 0.6 g of the drug; blood examination showed that he had a leukaemia, of which he died approximately 4 months later (Perers & Sjöberg, 1966).

(b) Epidemiological studies

Fraumeni (1967) conducted a follow-up study of 25 patients who developed bone-marrow depression following phenylbutazone therapy. Eighteen patients recovered within 2 weeks to 4 years, 4 were still under care at the time of the report and 3 died within 2 weeks to 2 years, 2 of aplastic anaemia and 1 of a myeloproliferative disorder, very probably a leukaemia.

4. Comments on Data Reported and Evaluation

4.1 Animal data

No data were available to the Working Group.

4.2 Human data

A number of cases of leukaemia were reported between 1960 and 1966 in subjects treated with phenylbutazone or oxyphenbutazone. The available evidence is, however, insufficient to substantiate the suggestion that use of phenylbutazone or oxyphenbutazone is related to subsequent developement of leukaemia.

5. References

American Society of Hospital Pharmacists (1961) American Hospital Formulary Service, Section 28:08, Washington DC

Anon. (1974) Production and imports of selected drugs and pharmaceuticals in India. Chemical Industry News (India), July

Bean, R.H.D. (1960) Phenylbutazone and leukaemia. A possible association. Brit. med. J., iv, 1552-1555

Bignami, M., Morpurgo, G., Pagliani, R., Carere, A., Conti, G. & Di Giuseppe, G. (1974) Non-disjunction and crossing-over induced by pharmaceutical drugs in Aspergillus nidulans. Mutation Res., 26, 159-170

British Pharmacopoeia Commission (1973) British Pharmacopoeia, London, HMSO, pp. 364-365

Bruce, R.B., Maynard, W.R., Jr, Dunning, L.K. (1974) Oxyphenbutazone and phenylbutazone determination in plasma and urine by GLC. J. pharm. Sci., 63, 446-448

Burns, J.J., Rose, R.K., Chenkin, T., Goldman, A., Schulert, A. & Brodie, B.B. (1953) The physiological disposition of phenylbutazone (Butazolidin) in man and a method for its estimation in biological material. J. Pharmacol. exp. Ther., 109, 346-357

Burns, J.J., Rose, R.K., Goodwin, S., Reichenthal, J., Horning, E.C. & Brodie, B.B. (1955) The metabolic fate of phenylbutazone (Butazolidin) in man. J. Pharmacol. exp. Ther., 113, 481-489

Cadman, E.F.B. & Limont, W. (1962) Phenylbutazone and leukaemia. Brit. med. J., i, 798

Cast, I.P. (1961) Phenylbutazone and leukaemia. Brit. med. J., iv, 1569-1570

Cavallito, C.J. (1968) Contributions of medicinal chemistry to medicine - from 1935. In: Jucker, E., ed, Progress in Drug Research, Vol. 12, Basel, Birkhäuser Verlag, p. 31

Chalmers, T.M. & McCarthy, D.D. (1964) Phenylbutazone therapy associated with leukaemia. Brit. med. J., i, 747

Chatterjea, J.B. (1964) Leukaemia and phenylbutazone. Brit. med. J., iv, 875

Dougan, L. & Woodliff, H.J. (1965) Acute leukaemia associated with phenylbutazone treatment: a review of the literature and report of a further case. Med. J. Austr., i, 217-219

Fraumeni, J.F., Jr (1967) Bone marrow depression induced by chloramphenicol or phenylbutazone. Leukemia and other sequelae. J. Amer. med. Ass., 201, 828-834

Garrett, J.V. (1961) Phenylbutazone and leukaemia. Brit. med. J., i, 53

Gebhart, E. & Wissmüller, H.F. (1973) Investigations on the effect of phenylbutazone on chromosomes and mitosis in the bone marrow of rats. Mutation Res., 17, 282-286

Golding, J.R., Hamilton, M.G. & Moody, H.E. (1965) Monocytic leukaemia and phenylbutazone. Brit. med. J., i, 1673

Häfliger, F. (1956) 1,2-Diphenyl-3,5-dioxopyrazolidines. US Patent 2,745,783, to J.R. Geigy A.G.

Hart, G.D. (1964) Leukaemia and phenylbutazone. Brit. med. J., ii, 569

Jähnchen, E. & Levy, G. (1972) Determination of phenylbutazone in plasma. Clin. Chem., 18, 984-986

Jensen, M.K. (1972) Phenylbutazone, chloramphenicol and mammalian chromosomes. Humangenetik, 17, 61-64

Jensen, M.K. & Roll, K. (1965) Phenylbutazone and leukaemia. Acta med. scand., 178, 505-513

Kastrup, E.K., ed. (1976) Facts and Comparisons, St Louis, Missouri, Facts and Comparisons, Inc., pp. 254d, 255

Kirsner, J.B. & Ford, H. (1955) Phenylbutazone (Butazolidin) - effect on basal gastric secretion and the production of gastroduodenal ulcerations in dogs. Gastroenterology, 29, 18-23

Knott, R.P. (1974) Drug therapy of gout. Pharmindex, November, p. 6

Krechniak, J., Foss, W. & Delag, G. (1972) Identification of butapirazol in biological material by thin-layer chromatography. Bromatol. Chem. Toksykol., 5, 443-447

Lawrence, A. (1960) Phenylbutazone and leukaemia. Brit. med. J., iv, 1736

Machemer, L. & Hess, R. (1971) Comparative dominant lethal studies with phenylbutazone, thio-TEPA and MMS in the mouse. Experientia, 27, 1050-1052

Machemer, L. & Hess, R. (1973) Induced dominant lethals in female mice: effects of triaziquone and phenylbutazone. Experientia, 29, 190-192

Magalhães, J.F. & Piros, M.G. (1973) Contribuição á espectrofotometria da fenilbutazona. Rev. Farm. Bioquim. Univ. Sao Paulo, 11, 41-50

Mauer, E.F. (1955) The toxic effects of phenylbutazone (Butazolidin): a review of literature and report of the twenty-third death following its use. New Engl. J. Med., 253, 404-410

McCann, J. & Ames, B.N. (1976) Detection of carcinogens as mutagens in the *Salmonella*/microsome test: assay of 300 chemicals: discussion. Proc. nat. Acad. Sci. (Wash.), 73, 950-954

McCann, J., Choi, E., Yamasaki, E. & Ames, B.N. (1975) Detection of carcinogens as mutagens in the *Salmonella*/microsome test: assay of 300 chemicals. Proc. nat. Acad. Sci. (Wash.), 72, 5135-5139

McGilveray, I.J., Midha, K.K., Brien, R. & Wilson, L. (1974) The assay of phenylbutazone in human plasma by a specific and sensitive gas-liquid chromatographic procedure. J. Chromat., 89, 17-22

Midha, K.K., McGilveray, I.J. & Charette, C. (1974) GLC determination of plasma concentration of phenylbutazone and its metabolite oxyphenbutazone. J. pharm. Sci., 63, 1234-1239

Müller, D. & Strasser, F.F. (1971) Comparative studies on the Chinese hamster bone marrow after treatment with phenylbutazone and cyclophosphamide. Mutation Res., 13, 377-382

National Formulary Board (1970) National Formulary XIII, Washington DC, American Pharmaceutical Association, pp. 510-512

Perers, D. & Sjöberg, S-G. (1966) Akut leukemi, leukemoid reaktion och leukocytos efter behandling med oxifenylbutazon. Läkartidningen, 63, 53-56

Pomazánska-Kołodziejska, T. (1972) Identification and determination of beta-diketones in drugs. I. Identification by thin-layer chromatography method. Acta pol. pharm., 29, 395-398

Pound, N.J. & Sears, R.W. (1975) Simultaneous determination of phenylbutazone and oxyphenbutazone in plasma by high-speed liquid chromatography. J. pharm. Sci., 64, 284-287

Pound, N.J., McGilveray, I.J. & Sears, R.W. (1974) Analysis of phenylbutazone in plasma by high-speed liquid chromatography. J. Chromat., 89, 23-30

Proksa, B., Molnár, L. & Szöcsová, H. (1974) Voltammetrische Bestimmung von Arzneimitteln aus der Gruppe 3,5-Dioxopyrazolidine. Pharm. Ind., 36, 805-806

Rathenberg, R. & Müller, D. (1972) Comparative cytogenetic studies of the influence of phenylbutazone and cyclophosphamide on spermatogenesis in the mouse. Agents and Actions, 2, 180-185

Saršúnová, M. & Kakáč, B. (1972) Dünnschichtchromatographie von Pyrazolon-
derivaten. Pharmazie, 27, 447-448

Stecher, P.G., ed. (1968) The Merck Index, 8th ed., Rahway, NJ, Merck &
Co., pp. 553 & 815

Stenzl, H. (1951) Derivatives of 3,5-dioxopyrazolidine. US Patent
2,562,830, to J.R. Geigy, A.G.

Stevenson, A.C., Bedford, J., Hill, A.G.S. & Hill, H.F.H. (1971) Chromosomal studies in patients taking phenylbutazone. Ann. Rheum. Dis.,
30, 487-500

Sunshine, I., ed. (1969) CRC Handbook of Analytical Toxicology, Cleveland,
Ohio, Chemical Rubber Co., pp. 84, 93

Szyszko, E. & Weglowska, W. (1974) Studies on decomposition of phenylbutazone solutions. II. Assays of phenylbutazone by alternating
current oscillopolarography. Acta pol. pharm., 31, 195-199

Tanimura, Y., Saitoh, Y., Nakagawa, F. & Suzuki, T. (1975) Determination
of phenylbutazone and its metabolites in plasma by a gas-liquid
chromatographic procedure. Chem. pharm. Bull. (Japan), 23, 651-658

Thorpe, G.J. (1964) Leukaemia and phenylbutazone. Brit. med. J., ii, 1707

US International Trade Commission (1976a) Synthetic Organic Chemicals, US
Production and Sales, 1974, USITC Publication 776, Washington DC,
US Government Printing Office, p. 105

US International Trade Commission (1976b) Imports of Benzenoid Chemicals
and Products, 1974, USITC Publication 762, Washington DC, US
Government Printing Office, p. 85

US Pharmacopeial Convention, Inc. (1975) The US Pharmacopeia, 19th rev.,
Rockville, Md, pp. 376-377

US Tariff Commission (1961) Synthetic Organic Chemicals, US Production and
Sales, 1960, TC Publication 34, Washington DC, US Government Printing
Office, p. 118

US Tariff Commission (1967) Synthetic Organic Chemicals, US Production and
Sales, 1965, TC Publication 206, Washington DC, US Government Printing
Office, p. 122

US Tariff Commission (1973) Imports of Benzenoid Chemicals and Products,
1972, TC Publication 601, Washington DC, US Government Printing
Office, pp. 86-87

US Tariff Commission (1974) Imports of Benzenoid Chemicals and Products,
1973, TC Publication 688, Washington DC, US Government Printing
Office, pp. 82-83

Watson, J.R., Matsui, F., Lawrence, R.C. & McConnell, P.M.J. (1973) The purity of phenylbutazone raw material and solid dosage forms as monitored by gas-liquid chromatography. *J. Chromat.*, 76, 141-147

Wissmüller, H.F. (1971) Untersuchungen über die cytogenetische Wirkung von Phenylbutazon an menschlichen Lymphocyten *in vitro*. *Arzneimittel-Forsch.*, 21, 1738-1750

Wissmüller, H. & Gebhart, E. (1970) Cytogenetic effects of Butazolidin in human leukocytes *in vitro*. *EMS Newslett.*, 3, 28-29

Woodbury, D.M. & Fingl, E. (1975) Analgesic-antipyretics, anti-inflammatory agents, and drugs employed in the therapy of gout. In: Goodman, L.S. & Gilman, A., eds, *The Pharmacological Basis of Therapeutics*, 5th ed., New York, Macmillan, pp. 339-341

Woodliff, H.J. & Dougan, L. (1964) Acute leukaemia associated with phenylbutazone treatment. *Brit. med. J.*, i, 744-746

PHENYTOIN AND PHENYTOIN SODIUM

1. Chemical and Physical Data

Phenytoin

1.1 Synonyms and trade names

Chem. Abstr. Reg. Serial No.: 57-41-0

Chem. Abstr. Name: 5,5-Diphenyl-2,4-imidazolidinedione

Diphenylhydantoin; 5,5-diphenylhydantoin; 5,5-diphenylimidazolidin-2,4-dione; DPH; phanantine; phenantoine

Aleviatin; Antisacer; Denyl; Didan-TDC-250; Difhydan; Dihycon; Di-Hydan; Dihydantoin; Di-Lan; Dilantin; Dilantine; Dillantin; Dintoina; Diphantoin; Diphedan; Diphenin; Diphenine; Diphentoine; Diphentyn; Enkefal; Epanutin; Epilan; Epinat; Eptoin; Gerot-Epilan-D; Hidantal; Hydantin; Lepitoin; Sodanton; Tacosal; Zentropil

1.2 Chemical formula and molecular weight

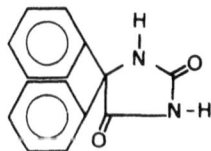

$$C_{15}H_{12}N_2O_2 \qquad \text{Mol. wt:}\ 252.3$$

1.3 Chemical and physical properties of the pure substance

From Stecher (1968), unless otherwise specified

(a) Description: Powder

(b) Melting-point: 295-298°C

(c) Spectroscopy data: λ_{max} 258 nm (E_1^1 = 28.1) in water (Weast, 1975); 264 and 257 nm (E_1^1 = 18.5 and 29.1) in methanol (Grasselli, 1973)

(d) Solubility: Practically insoluble in water; soluble in ethanol (1.7 g/100 ml) and in acetone (3.3 g/100 ml)

1.4 Technical products and impurities

Various national and international pharmacopoeias give specifications for the purity of phenytoin in pharmaceutical products. For example, phenytoin is available in the US as a USP grade containing 98.5-100.5% active ingredient on a dried basis with a maximum of 0.002% heavy metals, and as 50 mg tablets that contain 93-107% of the stated amount of phenytoin (US Pharmacopeial Convention, Inc., 1975). Oral suspensions of 6, 20 or 25 mg phenytoin per ml of a suitable medium are also available and contain 90-110% of the stated amount of phenytoin (National Formulary Board, 1970). Sustained release capsules of 50, 100, 125 or 250 mg phenytoin are also obtainable (Kastrup, 1975).

Phenytoin sodium

1.1 Synonyms and trade names

Chem. Abstr. Reg. Serial No.: 630-93-3

Chem. Abstr. Name: 5,5-Diphenyl-2,4-imidazolidinedione, monosodium salt

Diphenylhydantoin sodium; 5,5-diphenylhydantoin sodium; diphenyl-hydantoin sodium salt; 5,5-diphenylhydantoin sodium salt; phenytoinum sodium; sodium diphenylhydantoin; sodium 5,5-diphenylhydantoin; sodium 5,5'-diphenylhydantoin; sodium diphenylhydantoinate; sodium 5,5-diphenylhydantoinate; sodium 5,5-diphenyl-2,4-imidazolidinedione; sodium phenytoin; soluble phenytoin

Alepsin; Antilepsin; Antisacer; Auranile; Citrullamon; Dantoin; Denyl; Difenin; Difetoin; Difhydan; Di-Hydan; Dihydantoin; Dilantin; Dilantin Sodium; Dintoina; Diphantoine; Diphedan; Diphenate; Diphenin; Diphentoin; Di-Phetine; Ditoin; Divulsan; Enkefal; Epamin; Epanutin; Epelin; Epifenyl; Epihydan; Epilan-D; Epilantin; Epinat; Eptoin; Fenantoin; Fenitoin; Fenytoine; Hidantal; Hydantin; Hydantoin; Hydantoinal; Idantoin; Idantoinal; Lepitoin; Minetoin; Novantoina; Novodiphenyl; Om-Hydantoine; Phenhydan; Saceril; SDPH; Sodanton; Solantoin; Solantyl; Sylantoic; Tacosal; Thilophenyt; Zentropil

1.2 Chemical formula and molecular weight

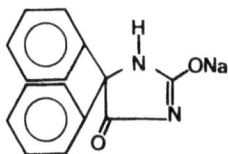

$$C_{15}H_{11}N_2NaO_2 \qquad \text{Mol. wt:} \quad 274.2$$

1.3 Chemical and physical properties of the pure substance

From Stecher (1968)

(a) Description: White powder

(b) Solubility: Soluble in water at pH > 11.7 (1.7 g/100 ml) and in ethanol (10 g/100 ml); insoluble in ether and chloroform

(c) Stability: Gradually absorbs carbon dioxide on exposure to air, liberating phenytoin

1.4 Technical products and impurities

Various national and international pharmacopoeias give specifications for the purity of phenytoin sodium in pharmaceutical products. For example, phenytoin sodium is available in the US as a USP grade containing 98.5-100.5% active ingredient on a dried basis with a maximum of 0.002% heavy metals. Capsules are available in 30 or 100 mg doses and contain 93-107% of the stated amount of phenytoin sodium. Sterile phenytoin sodium suitable for parenteral use is available in 100 or 250 mg doses in solution containing 90 115% of the stated amount (US Pharmacopeial Convention, Inc., 1975). Phenytoin sodium is available in powder form in 1, 4 or 16 oz doses (Kastrup, 1975).

In the UK, preparations contain 98.5-101% active ingredient on a dried basis and 92.5-107.5% of the stated amount of active ingredient in tablets (British Pharmacopoeia Commission, 1973).

2. Production, Use, Occurrence and Analysis

For important background information on this section, see preamble, p. 15.

2.1 Production and Use

(a) Production

A method of preparing phenytoin was patented in the US in 1946 (Henze, 1946). In one commercially used method, benzaldehyde is converted to benzoin with sodium cyanide followed by oxidation with nitric acid to benzil; this is heated with urea in aqueous ethanolic potassium hydroxide and acidified to give phenytoin. In another method, phenytoin is obtained by heating urea with benzilic acid in acetic anhydride (Smith, 1966).

In a method of preparing phenytoin sodium, reported by Biltz in 1911, benzil was condensed with urea followed by treatment with sodium hydroxide (Stecher, 1968). This method is still used currently, in addition to a similar method which involves the following steps: benzaldehyde is converted to benzoin using sodium cyanide, followed by oxidation with nitric acid to give benzil; this is heated with urea in the presence of ethanolic sodium ethoxide or isopropoxide to give phenytoin sodium (Smith, 1966; Swinyard, 1975).

Commercial production of phenytoin was first reported in the US in 1946 (US Tariff Commission, 1948); only one US company reported production (see preamble, p. 15) in 1974 (US International Trade Commission, 1976a). US imports of phenytoin through the principal customs districts were 900 kg in 1972 (US Tariff Commission, 1973), 550 kg in 1973 (US Tariff Commission, 1974) and 2,400 kg in 1974 (US International Trade Commission, 1976b).

Commercial production of phenytoin sodium was first reported in the US in 1938 (US Tariff Commission, 1939); only one US company reported production (see preamble, p. 15) in 1974 (US International Trade Commission, 1976a). US imports of phenytoin sodium were 1,500 kg in 1972 and in 1973 (US Tariff Commission, 1973, 1974) and 6,700 kg in 1974 (US International Trade Commission, 1976b).

No evidence was found that phenytoin is produced commercially in Japan. In 1975, 1,250 kg of this drug were imported; approximately 95% was converted into the sodium salt, and only 5% was used directly as an antiepileptic agent. Commercial production of phenytoin sodium was begun in 1951. In 1975, one company produced about 1300 kg, of which about 1100 kg were used within the country.

Annual production of phenytoin and of phenytoin sodium in western Europe is estimated to be less than 1000 kg. Benelux, the Federal Republic of Germany and Italy are believed to be the major producing countries.

(b) Use

Phenytoin and phenytoin sodium are used largely in the treatment of grand mal and psychomotor seizures, often in combination with phenobarbital or other anticonvulsants. The oral dosage for adults and children over six years of age is initially 100 mg 3 times per day and can gradually be increased by 100 mg every two to four weeks until the desired response is obtained. Maintenance dosages usually range from 300 to 600 mg daily. Maintenance dosages for children under six are usually 3 to 10 mg/kg bw per day (American Society of Hospital Pharmacists, 1969).

Phenytoin sodium is also used for the control of status epilepticus. It is preferably administered intravenously, but can be administered intramuscularly if necessary. It can also be used for the prophylactic control of seizures in neurosurgery. It is administered intramuscularly during surgery and is continued during the post-operative period (Kastrup, 1975).

Phenytoin and phenytoin sodium have been proposed for use as cardiac depressants (anti-arrhythmic). The oral dose is usually 100 mg 2 to 4 times per day. An intravenous dose of 50 to 100 mg of the sodium salt is repeated every ten to fifteen minutes as necessary up to a total maximum dose of 10 to 15 mg/kg bw (US Pharmacopeial Convention, Inc., 1975).

Phenytoin has been used in the treatment of chorea or Parkinson's syndrome to control involuntary movements. Its use has been investigated for the treatment of trigeminal neuralgia, migraine, polyneuritis of pregnancy, acute alcoholism and certain psychoses (American Society of Hospital Pharmacists, 1969). Phenytoin sodium has also been suggested for use in the treatment of migraine, trigeminal neuralgia and certain psychoses. However, these uses are not yet approved by the US Food and Drug Administration (Swinyard, 1975).

Total US sales of phenytoin for use in human medicine are estimated to be less than 78,000 kg annually.

Phenytoin is used in veterinary medicine to control epileptiform convulsions in dogs (Swinyard, 1975). Phenytoin sodium has also been recommended as an anticonvulsant for dogs (Stecher, 1968).

2.2 Occurrence

Phenytoin and phenytoin sodium are not known to occur in nature.

2.3 Analysis

Methods of assay of phenytoin that meet regulatory requirements for pharmaceutical products are usually based on non-aqueous titrations; those for phenytoin sodium are usually based on gravimetric methods.

A collaborative study investigated a column chromatographic method to separate phenytoin sodium in capsules followed by direct ultraviolet quantitation (Cunningham *et al.*, 1972).

A gas chromatographic method can determine phenytoin in serum in the range of 0.5-8.00 μg/ml (Brien & Inaba, 1974; Chin *et al.*, 1972). Another gas chromatographic method has been developed to determine phenytoin as its alkyl derivatives after flash-heater alkylation with tetraalkyl (C_1-C_7) ammonium hydroxides (Giovanniello & Pecci, 1976; Pecci & Giovanniello, 1975). Comparisons have been made of gas chromatographic methods for the determination of phenytoin in serum with a spectrophotometric method (Janz & Schmidt, 1974) and with an enzymatic immunoassay method (Booker & Darcey, 1975). A spin immunoassay determination of phenytoin in serum has been reported to have a minimum sensitivity of 20-30 nmol (Montgomery *et al.*, 1975).

Thin-layer chromatographic analyses of phenytoin can be made in pharmaceutical preparations (Prelini & Gerosa, 1975) and in blood and urine (Pippenger *et al.*, 1969).

High-pressure liquid chromatographic methods use UV spectrophotometric detection to determine phenytoin and phenobarbital in plasma (Atwell *et al.*, 1975), phenytoin and its *para*-hydroxylated metabolites in plasma (Albert *et al.*, 1973), phenytoin in blood (Gauchel *et al.*, 1973) and phenytoin, phenobarbital and primidone in blood (Kabra *et al.*, 1976). The limit of detection of these methods is in the order of 1 μg/ml.

A mass fragmentographic determination of phenytoin and its metabolite 5-(4-hydroxyphenyl)-5-phenylhydantoin in human plasma has a limit of detection of 0.01 μg/ml (Hoppel *et al.*, 1976).

An improved UV spectrophotometric method for the microdetermination of phenytoin in blood (Saitoh *et al.*, 1973) and a simplified fluorimetric method for its determination in plasma (Dill *et al.*, 1976) have been reported. A phosphorescence spectrometry method for determination of phenytoin in blood has a detection limit of 0.05 μg/ml (Morrison & O'Donnell, 1974).

A complexometric determination of phenytoin has also been reported (Hentrich & Pfeifer, 1967).

The methods of analysis for phenytoin in biological samples would, in principle, also be applicable to phenytoin sodium.

3. Biological Data Relevant to the Evaluation of Carcinogenic Risk to Man

3.1 Carcinogenicity and related studies in animals

(a) Oral administration

Mouse: Groups of 2-3-month old female C57BL, C3H/F or SJL/J mice, 48 animals per group, were fed phenytoin sodium at a dose level of 60 mg/kg bw/day in a liquid diet for 168 days. Three of 24 C57BL mice surviving 10 months developed thymic lymphomas, whereas no pathologic lesions were found in 48 controls. Three of 24 C3H/F female mice surviving 10 months developed localized thymic lymphomas, whereas no pathologic lesions were found in 48 controls (P=0.03). Six of 42 SJL/J mice autopsied after the 4th month had generalized lymphomas. After 8 or more months, 48 SJL/J controls showed proliferative atypical reticulum-cells but no lymphomas (Krüger *et al.*, 1972).

Rat: No tumours were observed in female or male Sprague-Dawley rats treated with high doses of phenytoin by gavage or in the diet and observed for periods of 6 to 13 months. Negative results were also obtained in female Holtzman rats given phenytoin in the diet and observed for 60 weeks (Griswold *et al.*, 1966, 1968; Morris *et al.*, 1969; Peraino *et al.*, 1975). No vesicular tumours were observed in male Long-Evans rats given phenytoin for one year, despite the presence of a surgically implanted foreign body in the vesicle. No tumours were seen in non-operated controls (McDonald, 1969) [These negative studies were inadequate in duration to be of value in assessing carcinogenic activity].

(b) Intraperitoneal administration

Mouse: Fifty random bred albino mice of both sexes (18-20 g) received daily i.p. injections of 0.6 mg/animal phenytoin suspended in water or in saline over 66 days (total, 57 injections or 34.2 mg/animal). No weight gain was observed, and 10 animals died during this period. The remaining 40 animals were observed for 9 months; 50 untreated controls were observed for 11 months. Ten treated mice developed tumours, comprising 4 thymic and 2 mesenteric lymphomas and 4 leukaemias. The leukaemias developed between 60 and 142 days and the lymphomas between 100 and 255 days. In controls, 1 thymic lymphoma and 1 lung adenoma were observed (Juhász *et al.*, 1968).

3.2 Other relevant biological data

(a) Experimental systems

The i.v. LD_{50} of phenytoin sodium in rabbits is 125 mg/kg bw (Stecher, 1968). Oral administration of phenytoin sodium to dogs produced higher plasma peak levels at earlier time periods than phenytoin (Glazko, 1972).

Phenytoin administered intraveneously to male Sprague-Dawley rats was found to accumulate to a considerable degree, immediately after adminis- tration, in the liver, kidney and salivary gland and at a slower rate and to a smaller degree in fat, muscle and brain (Noach *et al.*, 1958). With continuous administration to ferrets, high concentrations were found in the oral mucosa as well as in the salivary gland (Steinberg *et al.*, 1973). Breakdown of ^{14}C-phenytoin in the liver of Sprague-Dawley rats first suggested that liver was the principal site of metabolism (Noach *et al.*,

1958), and its hepatic metabolism has been demonstrated in isolated perfused livers of rats of that strain (Gerber *et al.*, 1971). Metabolites are excreted in bile (Gerber *et al.*, 1973) and in urine (Chang *et al.*, 1972).

The principal metabolites were formed by hydroxylation of one of the phenyl rings (Butler, 1957) in the *para* position in rats (Chang *et al.*, 1972) and in the *meta* position in dogs (Atkinson *et al.*, 1970) and were excreted in the urine as glucuronides (Atkinson *et al.*, 1970; Chang *et al.*, 1972; Maynert, 1960).

In addition, 5-(3,4-dihydroxy-1,5-cyclohexadien-1-yl)-5-phenylhydantoin has been identified in rat and monkey urine (Chang *et al.*, 1970). In rat urine, the diphenolic metabolite 5-(3,4-dihydroxyphenyl)-5-phenylhydantoin (Borga *et al.*, 1972) and its methoxylated derivative, 5-(4-hydroxy-3-methoxy-phenyl)-5-phenylhydantoin, are present as glucuronide conjugates (Chang *et al.*, 1972). The glucuronic acid conjugates of 5-(3,4-dihydroxyphenyl)-5-phenylhydantoin and 5-(3-methoxy-4-hydroxyphenyl)-5-phenylhydantoin were identified in rat bile (Gerber *et al.*, 1973) as well as 5,5-bis(4-hydroxy-phenyl)hydantoin (Thompson *et al.*, 1976).

A single intragastric dose of phenytoin to pregnant Sprague-Dawley rats was transferred to the foetuses and was concentrated more in the kidney than in the liver, in contrast to the situation in adult rats (Gabler & Falace, 1970). Transplacental transport has been documented in mice (Stevens & Harbison, 1974; Waddell & Mirkin, 1972), rats (Mirkin, 1971; Stevens & Harbison, 1974), hamsters (Stevens & Harbison, 1974), goats (Shoeman *et al.*, 1972) and monkeys (Gabler & Hubbard, 1972).

A/Jax mice were injected subcutaneously with 12.5, 25 or 50 mg/kg bw phenytoin sodium at various times from days 9-15 of pregnancy; the 50 mg/kg bw dose produced cleft palates in 26-43% of the offspring (Massey, 1966).

Pregnant Swiss-Webster and A/J mice were injected subcutaneously with 50 mg/kg bw phenytoin sodium on days 7-9 or 11-13 of gestation. Treatment during late gestation induced significant increases in the incidence of cleft palates in the offspring of Swiss-Webster (15%) and A/J mice (31%) (Gibson & Becker, 1968). The teratogenicity of phenytoin has been confirmed in other experiments in mice (Elshove, 1969; Harbison & Becker, 1969;

Marsh & Fraser, 1973;   Sullivan & McElhatton, 1975), rats (Harbison & Becker, 1972;   Mercier-Parot & Tuchmann-Duplessis, 1974) and monkeys (Wilson, 1973).

After oral treatment of rats with 250 mg/kg bw daily for the first 5 days of gestation, bone-marrow cells had 26% abnormal metaphases compared with 8% in controls (and accumulation of metaphases was also observed) (Caratzali & Roman, 1971;   Roman & Caratzali, 1971).

Negative results have been reported in the dominant lethal test in mice after 115 or 145 mg/kg bw phenytoin sodium were administered by i.p. injection (Epstein *et al.*, 1972).

(b)   Man

A single oral dose of phenytoin sodium produced higher blood levels of the sodium salt than did phenytoin (Dill *et al.*, 1956).

The principal adverse reaction to phenytoin is gingival hyperplasia (Hassell *et al.*, 1976;   Kapur *et al.*, 1973).   In addition, hepatic necrosis (Lee *et al.*, 1976) and a reduction in the number of peripheral blood lymphocytes (Brandt & Nilsson, 1976) have been reported;   atypical lymph node hyperplasia ('pseudolymphoma') may also occur (see section 3.3).

Following a single oral dose of phenytoin sodium, 5-(*para*-hydroxyphenyl)-5-phenylhydantoin and a 10-fold greater level of its glucuronide were present in plasma (Albert *et al.*, 1974).   Urine samples from individuals receiving phenytoin contain 5-13% of the hydroxylated metabolite as 5-(*meta*-hydroxyphenyl)-5-phenylhydantoin (Atkinson *et al.*, 1970).   Other urinary metabolites are 5-(3,4-dihydroxy-1,5-cyclohexadien-1-yl)-5-phenylhydantoin (Horning *et al.*, 1971), 5-(3,4-dihydroxyphenyl)-5-phenylhydantoin (Borga *et al.*, 1972) and 5,5-bis-(4-hydroxyphenyl)hydantoin (Thompson *et al.*, 1976).

A possible association between maternal epilepsy, anticonvulsant drugs (mainly phenytoin and phenobarbital) and congenital malformations in offspring was reported by Meadow (1968).   In two reports, a total of 38 children born to mothers who took anticonvulsants, including phenytoin, throughout pregnancy revealed a similar constellation of malformations suggesting a syndrome involving the lip and palate, cardiovascular system and skeletal abnormalities (limb, skull, face) (Meadow, 1968, 1970). Subsequent case reports of epileptic women treated during pregnancy with phenytoin and phenobarbital have described affected infants with similar abnormalities (Aase, 1974; Anderson, 1976; Barr *et al.*, 1974; Dabee *et al.*, 1975; Goodman *et al.*, 1976; Loughnan *et al.*, 1973; Pettifor & Benson, 1975).

In a retrospective study of epileptic mothers in the Federal Republic of Germany, 262 pregnancies were accompanied by continuous treatment with phenytoin and barbiturates; five malformations were found among the offspring, to give a rate of 2.2%, which was not considered to be increased over that of the general population (Janz & Fuchs, 1964).

In 51 pregnancies identified from US hospital records over the period 1960-1970 occurring in 42 epileptic patients, phenytoin was administered alone or with mysoline in 7 pregnancies and with phenobarbital in 44 pregnancies, throughout pregnancy; 3 congenital abnormalities occurred (5.8%). Although no anomalies were found in 50 matched pregnancies, the effect was not considered to be statistically significant (Watson & Spellacy, 1971).

In the UK, 168 epileptic women treated with phenytoin, phenobarbital or other anticonvulsant drugs were identified from the neurology departments of two general hospitals. These women had experienced 365 pregnancies, during which phenytoin alone or in combination was given during 192 pregnancies and phenobarbital alone or in combination during 240 pregnancies. Seventeen of the 365 infants had malformations, compared with 7 of 483 controls and 0 of 62 offspring of epileptic women not taking medication. The calculated risk was two to three times greater than normal (Speidel & Meadow, 1972).

During 1969 and 1970, 7,896 women gave birth at a single London hospital, and 192 of the infants had malformations, to give a rate of 2.44%. In this group, 22 epileptic mothers had taken anticonvulsant drugs throughout pregnancy. Two of the children born to mothers who had taken phenytoin and phenobarbital in one case and phenytoin and other drugs in the other case had cleft palate and/or hare lip, an incidence of 9%, whereas only 0.13% of the infants born to non-epileptic mothers were so affected (South, 1972).

In the US, the outcome of 50,897 pregnancies selected from patients attending 12 hospitals between 1959 and 1965 were examined. The congenital malformation rate for a wide range of defects, including cleft lip and cleft palate, was 6.12% among births to 98 epileptic mothers who took phenytoin regularly during the first four months of pregnancy. The rate was significantly higher than that of 2.45% among children born to women with no convulsive disorder. The abnormality rate among babies born to 101 women with convulsive disorders but who did not receive phenytoin was 2.97%, which is not significantly different from normal (Monson et al., 1973).

In Cardiff, 31,877 infants born between 1965 and 1971 were studied; 245 mothers in this series had a history of epilepsy. Among the 111 births to epileptic mothers not on anticonvulsant therapy, the malformation rate was 2.7%, compared to 2.8% of infants in the total population. In contrast, 6.7% of 134 infants born to mothers receiving anticonvulsant therapy had malformations: 1/53 children whose mothers had received phenobarbital alone, 2/9 children whose mothers had received phenytoin alone and 6/60 children whose mothers had received phenobarbital and phenytoin during pregnancy (Lowe, 1973)

In US Air Force hospitals between 1965 and 1971, among the children born to 410 epileptic mothers almost certainly exposed to anticonvulsant therapy during pregnancy, from a population of 347,097 liveborn infants, there was a two-fold increase in the risk for all malformations and a five- to six-fold increase for cleft lip and/or palate (Niswander & Wertelecki, 1973). In a survey in Northern Ireland, the risk to infants born to epileptic mothers taking anticonvulsant drugs, mainly phenytoin and phenobarbital and other drugs, was 6.4% compared with a malformation rate of 3.8% for all live and stillbirths in the province. There was a 7-fold increase in the risk of cleft lip with or without cleft palate (1.8% compared with 0.22%) (Millar & Nevin, 1973).

In the Oxford Record Linkage Study, of live babies born between 1966 and 1970 to epileptic mothers, 17/217 (7.8%) had congenital abnormalities

212

at birth compared with 21/649 (3.2%) of the controls matched for civil status, social class, maternal age, parity, hospital and year of delivery. Subsequently, the rates rose to 13.8% (30/217) for babies of epileptic mothers and 5.6% (36/649) for those in the control group [This may be due to the longer observation period and to the inclusion of different types of malformations, which could have been considered to be congenital before]. Maternal phenobarbital ingestion alone did not account for an increased incidence of defects (2/41, 4.9%) over that in infants of mothers not taking drugs (2/19, 10.5%), but when given in combination with phenytoin the proportion of infants with defects is more than doubled (11/50, 21%). The incidence of defects among infants of mothers taking phenytoin alone (5/33, 15.2%), while higher than that among infants of mothers taking phenobarbital alone, is lower than that among infants of mothers taking phenytoin in combination with phenobarbital (Fedrick, 1973).

In Scotland between 1965 and 1967, a prospective study of 15,181 pregnancy outcomes, including abortions and including 48 epileptic mothers, revealed 452 with malformations, of which 30 had hare lip and/or cleft palate. None of these were associated with epilepsy or anticonvulsant therapy in the mother. It was concluded that any causative relationship between anticonvulsant therapy and teratogenic effects would require a larger study (Kuenssberg & Knox, 1973).

A study of pregnancies followed in a single US clinic included 284 births to 138 epileptic mothers between 1939 and 1972. Of 141 births to mothers taking anticonvulsants during the first trimester, 10 infants had malformations; of 56 births to epileptics not taking medication, 1 infant had a malformation; and in 26 births to epileptic mothers in remission no malformations were seen. The association of cleft palate and heart malformations with anticonvulsant usage was similar in 28 patients treated with phenobarbital alone and in 24 patients treated with phenytoin alone (Annegers *et al.*, 1974).

Barry & Danks (1974) reported that in Australia between 1967 and 1972, 10/39 infants born to mothers treated with phenytoin and barbiturates during pregnancy had congenital abnormalities. No congenital abnormalities occurred in children of mothers treated with barbiturates alone, whereas they occurred in 2/8 children of mothers treated with phenytoin.

The teratogenicity of phenytoin has also been designated as the foetal hydantoin syndrome (Hanson, 1976; Hanson & Smith, 1975) (see also monograph on phenobarbital and phenobarbital sodium, p. 157).

In vitro treatment of human peripheral leucocytes with concentrations of 50-100 µg/ml phenytoin produced chromosome abnormalities (Muñiz *et al.*, 1969). Negative results have also been obtained with similar concentrations (Alving *et al.*, 1976; Bishun *et al.*, 1975; Stenchever & Jarvis, 1971).

A weak colchicine-like effect on metaphase arrest in cultured human lymphocytes has been observed *in vitro* with concentrations of 3.6×10^{-4} M. In the same study, the metabolite 5-(4-hydroxyphenyl)-5-phenylhydantoin was 3 times more potent (MacKinney *et al.*, 1975). A preliminary report indicated that both phenytoin and the metabolite interfere with microtubule formation *in vitro* (MacKinney & Vyas, 1975).

Chromosomes in cultured leucocytes from 7 epileptic patients receiving phenytoin sodium showed no abnormalities (Muñiz *et al.*, 1969). Chromosomal abnormalities were, however, reported by Neuhauser *et al.* (1970). In a study of leucocyte cultures from 32 mothers taking anticonvulsants, the average increase in chromosomal abnormalities was 17% in those of all 5 women taking only phenytoin, whereas only 5% was seen in cultures from 32 controls; leucocytes of 4 children born to mothers receiving phenytoin only also had an increased number of mitotic abnormalities (Grosse *et al.*, 1972).

3.3 Case reports and epidemiological studies

(a) Case reports

Of 7 patients originally described by Saltzstein & Ackerman (1959) as developing pseudolymphomas following phenytoin and/or phenobarbital treatment, two died, one from multiple myeloma with an unknown survival time after diagnosis, and another from malignant lymphoma within 4 years (Harrington *et al.*, 1962).

Of 6 patients receiving phenytoin alone or with phenobarbital, 3 were reported to have developed Hodgkin's disease, 2, lymphosarcomas and 1, a reticulum-cell sarcoma (Hyman & Sommers, 1966).

214

Numerous case reports have described lymphomas (Bichel, 1975; Brown, 1971; Gams et al., 1968; Jungi et al., 1975; Rausing & Trell, 1971; Sorrell & Forbes, 1975; Tashima & de los Santos, 1974) and leukaemias (Wildhack, 1973) occurring in patients treated with phenytoin.

Two cases of neuroblastoma, a 3-year old girl and a 7-day old boy, have been reported in the foetal hydantoin syndrome. Both mothers had taken anticonvulsants (phenytoin and phenobarbital) since girlhood because of epilepsy (Pendergrass & Hanson, 1976; Sherman & Roizen, 1976).

(b) Epidemiological studies

The records of 85 persons dying with malignant lymphomas during the period 1958 to 1968 at a single US hospital were reviewed for a history of phenytoin therapy. Four of the 85 were epileptics who received phenytoin sodium alone or phenobarbital. The occurrence of epilepsy was estimated to be 1 in 200 in the general population and in the necropsy group in this hospital, 1 in 400. Therefore, four lymphomas in 85 autopsies was 10 times the expected incidence (Anthony, 1970).

In 300 patients from a single US medical centre with malignant lymphomas, 7 were found to have a history of antiepileptic phenytoin therapy. Since only 1 in 300 individuals in the general population takes anticonvulsant drugs, this was considered to be a significant association (Charlton & Lunsford, 1971).

In a Danish hospital, 9,136 cases of epilepsy treated with phenytoin, phenobarbital or primidone during the period 1933 to 1962 were reviewed for the incidence of neoplasms. There was no increase in the incidence of neoplasms of the lymph and blood systems in the group of epileptics as compared with that in the general population (For a discussion on the incidence of liver tumours, see monograph on phenobarbital and phenobarbital sodium, p. 157). In patients treated for more than 10 years, tumours of brain and nervous system were observed in 10 males (expected 3.5) and in 6 females (expected 2.9) (Clemmesen et al., 1974) (see also 'General Remarks on Substances Considered', pp. 24-25).

A review of 516 cases of malignant lymphomas treated in a radiation centre during the period 1968 to 1972 revealed that 8 patients (1.6%) had

had prolonged treatment with phenytoin. Only 2 of 516 tumour-free individuals (0.4%) interviewed in connection with other epidemiologic studies had had phenytoin therapy. Three of 516 patients (0.6%), matched to within 5 years of age at diagnosis of cancers other than lymphoma, had received phenytoin therapy. Therefore, the excess risk of malignant lymphoma was concluded to be two- to three-fold for patients receiving phenytoin (Li *et al.*, 1975).

4. Comments on Data Reported and Evaluation

4.1 Animal data

Phenytoin and its sodium salt are carcinogenic in mice following their intraperitoneal injection and oral administration, respectively: they produced lymphomas and leukaemias. Studies in which rats were given phenytoin by oral administration were of too short duration to allow an evaluation to be made.

4.2 Human data

An association has been observed in epileptic patients between the occurrence of lymphomas and long-term anticonvulsant therapy in which phenytoin alone or in combination with other anticonvulsants such as phenobarbital were given (see also monograph on phenobarbital and phenobarbital sodium, p. 157).

5. References

Aase, J.M. (1974) Anticonvulsant drugs and congenital abnormalities. Amer. J. Dis. Child., 127, 758

Albert, K.S., Hallmark, M.R., Carroll, M.E. & Wagner, J.G. (1973) Quantitative separation of diphenylhydantoin and its *para*-hydroxylated metabolites by high-performance liquid chromatography. Res. Comm. chem. Path. Pharmacol., 6, 845-854

Albert, K.S., Hallmark, M.R., Sakmar, E., Weidler, D.J. & Wagner, J.G. (1974) Plasma concentrations of diphenylhydantoin, its *para*-hydroxylated metabolite, and corresponding glucuronide in man. Res. Comm. chem. Path. Pharmacol., 9, 463-469

Alving, J., Jensen, M.K. & Meyer, H. (1976) Diphenylhydantoin and chromosome morphology in man and rat. A negative report. Mutation Res., 40, 173-176

American Society of Hospital Pharmacists (1969) American Hospital Formulary Service, Section 28:12, Washington DC

Anderson, R.C. (1976) Cardiac defects in children of mothers receiving anticonvulsant therapy during pregnancy. J. Pediat., 89, 318-319

Annegers, J.F., Elveback, L.R., Hauser, W.A. & Kurland, L.T. (1974) Do anticonvulsants have a teratogenic effect? Arch. Neurol., 31, 364-373

Anthony, J.J. (1970) Malignant lymphoma associated with hydantoin drugs. Arch. Neurol., 22, 450-454

Atkinson, A.J., Jr, MacGee, J., Strong, J., Garteiz, D. & Gaffney, T.E. (1970) Identification of 5-*meta*-hydroxyphenyl-5-phenylhydantoin as a metabolite of diphenylhydantoin. Biochem. Pharmacol., 19, 2483-2491

Atwell, S.H., Green, V.A. & Haney, W.G. (1975) Development and evaluation of method for simultaneous determination of phenobarbital and diphenylhydantoin in plasma by high-pressure liquid chromatography. J. pharm. Sci., 64, 806-809

Barr, M., Jr, Poznanski, A.K. & Schmickel, R.D. (1974) Digital hypoplasia and anticonvulsants during gestation: a teratogenic syndrome? J. Pediat., 84, 254-256

Barry, J.E. & Danks, D.M. (1974) Anticonvulsants and congenital abnormalities. Lancet, ii, 48-49

Bichel, J. (1975) Hydantoin derivatives and malignancies of the haemopoietic system. Acta med. scand., 198, 327-328

Bishun, N.P., Smith, N.S. & Williams, D.C. (1975) Chromosomes and anticonvulsant drugs. Mutation Res., 28, 141-143

Booker, H.E. & Darcey, B.A. (1975) Enzymatic immunoassay vs. gas/liquid chromatography for determination of phenobarbital and diphenylhydantoin in serum. Clin. Chem., 21, 1766-1768

Borgå, O., Garle, M. & Gutová, M. (1972) Identification of 5-(3,4-dihydroxyphenyl)-5-phenylhydantoin as a metabolite of 5,5-diphenylhydantoin (phenytoin) in rats and man. Pharmacology, 7, 129-137

Brandt, L. & Nilsson, P.G. (1976) Lymphocytopenia in patients treated with phenytoin. Lancet, i, 308

Brien, J.F. & Inaba, T. (1974) Determination of low levels of 5,5-diphenylhydantoin in serum by gas-liquid chromatography. J. Chromat., 88, 265-270

British Pharmacopoeia Commission (1973) British Pharmacopoeia, London, HMSO, p. 367

Brown, J.M. (1971) Drug-associated lymphadenopathies with special reference to the Reed-Sternberg cell. Med. J. Austr., i, 375-378

Butler, T.C. (1957) The metabolic conversion of 5,5-diphenyl hydantoin to 5-(p-hydroxyphenyl)-5-phenyl hydantoin. J. Pharmacol. exp. Ther., 119, 1-11

Caratzali, A. & Roman, I.C. (1971) Action de la diphényl-hydantoïne sur les chromosomes. C.R. Acad. Sci. (Paris), Série D, 272, 663-664

Chang, T., Savory, A. & Glazko, A.J. (1970) A new metabolite of 5,5-diphenylhydantoin (dilantin). Biochem. biophys. Res. Comm., 38, 444-449

Chang, T., Okerholm, R.A. & Glazko, A.J. (1972) A 3-0-methylated catechol metabolite of diphenylhydantoin (dilantin) in rat urine. Res. Comm. chem. Path. Pharmacol., 4, 13-23

Charlton, M.H. & Lunsford, D. (1971) Le sostanze di idantoina come possibili cause del linfoma maligno. Minerva med., 62, 2185

Chin, D., Fastlich, E. & Davidow, B. (1972) The determination of 5,5-diphenylhydantoin (dilantin) in serum by gas chromatography. J. Chromat., 71, 545-548

Clemmesen, J., Fuglsang-Frederiksen, V. & Plum, C.M. (1974) Are anti-convulsants oncogenic? Lancet, i, 705-707

Cunningham, C.G., Brunner, C.A. & Levine, J. (1972) Collaborative study of a chromatographic method for sodium diphenylhydantoin in capsules. J. Ass. off. analyt. Chem., 55, 170-172

Dabee, V., Hart, A.G. & Hurley, R.M. (1975) Teratogenic effects of diphenylhydantoin. Canad. med. Ass. J., 112, 75-76

Dill, W.A., Kazenko, A., Wolf, L.M. & Glazko, A.J. (1956) Studies on 5,5'-diphenylhydantoin (dilantin) in animals and man. J. Pharmacol. exp. Ther., 118, 270-279

Dill, W.A., Leung, A., Kinkel, A.W. & Glazko, A.J. (1976) Simplified fluorometric assay for diphenylhydantoin in plasma. Clin. Chem., 22, 908-911

Elshove, J. (1969) Cleft palate in the offspring of female mice treated with phenytoin. Lancet, ii, 1074

Epstein, S.S., Arnold, E., Andrea, J., Bass, W. & Bishop, Y. (1972) Detection of chemical mutagens by the dominant lethal assay in the mouse. Toxicol. appl. Pharmacol., 23, 288-325

Fedrick, J. (1973) Epilepsy and pregnancy: a report from the Oxford Record Linkage Study. Brit. med. J., ii, 442-448

Gabler, W.L. & Falace, D. (1970) The distribution and metabolism of dilantin in non-pregnant, pregnant and fetal rats. Arch. int. Pharmacodyn., 184, 45-58

Gabler, W.L. & Hubbard, G.L. (1972) The distribution of 5,5-diphenyl-hydantoin (DPH) and its metabolites in maternal and fetal rhesus monkey tissues. Arch. int. Pharmacodyn., 200, 222-230

Gams, R.A., Neal, J.A. & Conrad, F.G. (1968) Hydantoin-induced pseudo-lymphoma. Ann. int. Med., 69, 557-568

Gauchel, G., Gauchel, F.D. & Birkofer, L. (1973) Eine Mikromethode zur Bestimmung von Diphenylhydantoin (Phenhydan) im Blut durch Flüssigkeits-Chromatographie mit hohen Eingangsdrucken. Z. klin. Chem. klin. Biochem., 11, 35-38

Gerber, N., Weller, W.L., Lynn, R., Rangno, R.E., Sweetman, B.J. & Bush, M.T. (1971) Study of dose-dependent metabolism of 5,5-diphenylhydantoin in the rat using new methodology for isolation and quantitation of metabolites in vivo and in vitro. J. Pharmacol. exp. Ther., 178, 567-579

Gerber, N., Seibert, R.A. & Thompson, R.M. (1973) Identification of a catechol glucuronide metabolite of 5,5-diphenylhydantoin (DPH) in rat bile by gas chromatography (GC) and mass spectrometry (MS). Res. Comm. chem. Path. Pharmacol., 6, 499-511

Gibson, J.E. & Becker, B.A. (1968) Teratogenic effects of diphenylhydantoin in Swiss-Webster and A/J mice. Proc. Soc. exp. Biol. (N.Y.), 128, 905-909

Giovanniello, T.J. & Pecci, J. (1976) Simultaneous isothermal determination of diphenylhydantoin and phenobarbital serum levels by gas-liquid chromatography following flash-heater hexylation. Clin. chim. acta, 67, 7-13

Glazko, A.J. (1972) Diphenylhydantoin. Pharmacology, 8, 163-177

Goodman, R.M., Katznelson, M.B-M., Hertz, M., Katznelson, D. & Rotem, Y. (1976) Congenital malformations in four siblings of a mother taking anticonvulsant drugs. Amer. J. Dis. Child., 130, 884-887

Grasselli, J.G., ed. (1973) CRC Atlas of Spectral Data and Physical Constants for Organic Compounds, Cleveland, Ohio, Chemical Rubber Co., p. B-604

Griswold, D.P., Jr, Casey, A.E., Weisburger, E.K., Weisburger, J.H., & Schabel, F.M., Jr (1966) On the carcinogenicity of a single intra-gastric dose of hydrocarbons, nitrosamines, aromatic amines, dyes, coumarins and miscellaneous chemicals in female Sprague-Dawley rats. Cancer Res., 26, 619-625

Griswold, D.P., Jr, Casey, A.E., Weisburger, E.K. & Weisburger, J.H. (1968) The carcinogenicity of multiple intragastric doses of aromatic and heterocyclic nitro or amino derivatives in young female Sprague-Dawley rats. Cancer Res., 28, 924-933

Grosse, K-P., Schwanitz, G., Rott, H-D. & Wissmüller, H.F. (1972) Chromo-somenuntersuchungen bei Behandlung mit Antikonvulsiva. Humangenetik, 16, 209-216

Hanson, J.W. (1976) Fetal hydantoin syndrome. Teratology, 13, 185-187

Hanson, J.W. & Smith, D.W. (1975) The fetal hydantoin syndrome. J. Pediat., 87, 285-290

Harbison, R.D. & Becker, B.A. (1969) Relation of dosage and time of administration of diphenylhydantoin to its teratogenic effect in mice. Teratology, 2, 305-311

Harbison, R.D. & Becker, B.A. (1972) Diphenylhydantoin teratogenicity in rats. Toxicol. appl. Pharmacol., 22, 193-200

Harrington, W.J., Tosteson, P.K., McAlister, W.H., Saltzstein, S.L., Brown, E., Restrepo, A., Fliedner, T.M., Loeb, V., Jr, Parker, B.M. & Kissane, J. (1962) Lymphoma or drug reaction occurring during hydantoin therapy for epilepsy. Amer. J. Med., 32, 286-297

Hassell, T.M., Page, R.C., Narayanan, A.S. & Cooper, C.G. (1976) Diphenyl-hydantoin (dilantin) gingival hyperplasia: drug-induced abnormality of connective tissue. Proc. nat. Acad. Sci. (Wash.), 73, 2909-2912

Hentrich, K. & Pfeifer, S. (1967) Komplexometrische Bestimmung von Phenytoin. Pharmazie, 22, 666-667

Henze, H.R. (1946) 5,5-Diarylhydantoins. US Patent 2,409,754, October 22, to Parke, Davis & Co.

Hoppel, C., Garle, M. & Elander, M. (1976) Mass fragmentographic determination of diphenylhydantoin and its main metabolite, 5-(4-hydroxyphenyl)-5-phenylhydantoin, in human plasma. J. Chromat., 116, 53-61

Horning, M.G., Stratton, C., Wilson, A., Horning, E.C. & Hill, R.M. (1971) Detection of 5-(3,4-dihydroxy-1,5-cyclohexadien-1-yl)-5-phenylhydantoin as a major metabolite of 5,5-diphenylhydantoin (dilantin) in the newborn human. Analyt. Lett., 4, 537-545

Hyman, G.A. & Sommers, S.C. (1966) The development of Hodgkin's disease and lymphoma during anticonvulsant therapy. Blood, 28, 416-427

Janz, D. & Fuchs, U. (1964) Sind antiepileptische Medikamente während der Schwangerschaft schädlich? Dtsch med. Wschr., 89, 241-243

Janz, D. & Schmidt, D. (1974) Comparison of spectrophotometric and gas-liquid chromatographic measurements of serum diphenylhydantoin concentrations in epileptic out-patients. J. Neurol., 207, 109-116

Juhász, J., Baló, J. & Szende, B. (1968) Experimental tumours developing upon the effect of diphenylhydantoin treatment. Magyar Onkol., 12, 39-44

Jungi, W.F., Senn, H.J., Stanisic, M. & Rösli, R. (1975) Maligne Lymphome nach jahrelanger Epilepsiebehandlung mit Hydantoinpräparaten? Schweiz. med. Wschr., 105, 1735-1737

Kabra, P.M., Gotelli, G., Stanfill, R. & Marton, L.J. (1976) Simultaneous measurement of phenobarbital, diphenylhydantoin, and primidone in blood by high-pressure liquid chromatography. Clin. Chem., 22, 824-827

Kapur, R.N., Girgis, S., Little, T.M. & Masotti, R.E. (1973) Diphenyl-hydantoin-induced gingival hyperplasia: its relationship to dose and serum level. Develop. Med. Child Neurol., 15, 483-487

Kastrup, E.K., ed. (1975) Facts and Comparisons, St Louis, Missouri, Facts and Comparisons, Inc., pp. 283e-283h, 284a-284b

Krüger, G., Harris, D. & Sussman, E. (1972) Effect of dilantin in mice. II. Lymphoreticular tissue atypia and neoplasia after chronic exposure. Z. Krebsforsch., 78, 290-302

Kuenssberg, E.V. & Knox, J.D.E. (1973) Teratogenic effect of anticonvulsants. Lancet, i, 198

Lee, T.J., Carney, C.N., Lapis, J.L., Higgins, T. & Fallon, H.J. (1976) Diphenylhydantoin-induced hepatic necrosis: a case study. Gastroenterology, 70, 422-424

Li, F.P., Willard, D.R., Goodman, R. & Vawter, G. (1975) Malignant lymphoma after diphenylhydantoin (dilantin) therapy. Cancer, 36, 1359-1362

Loughnan, P.M., Gold, H. & Vance, J.C. (1973) Phenytoin teratogenicity in man. Lancet, i, 70-72

Lowe, C.R. (1973) Congenital malformations among infants born to epileptic women. Lancet, i, 9-10

MacKinney, A. & Vyas, R. (1975) The effect of hydantoins on mitosis and microtubules. Clin. Res., 23, 384A

MacKinney, A.A., Vyas, R. & Lee, S.S. (1975) The effect of parahydroxy-lation of diphenylhydantoin on metaphase accumulation. Proc. Soc. exp. Biol. (N.Y.), 149, 371-375

Marsh, L. & Fraser, F.C. (1973) Studies on dilantin-induced cleft palate in mice. Teratology, 7, A-23

Massey, K.M. (1966) Teratogenic effects of diphenylhydantoin sodium. J. oral Ther. Pharmacol., 2, 380-385

Maynert, E.W. (1960) The metabolic fate of diphenylhydantoin in the dog, rat and man. J. Pharmacol. exp. Ther., 130, 275-284

McDonald, D.F. (1969) Lack of effect of diphenylhydantoin ingestion on vesical transitional epithelium in the rat. J. surg. Oncol., 1, 77-79

Meadow, S.R. (1968) Anticonvulsant drugs and congenital abnormalities. Lancet, ii, 1296

Meadow, S.R. (1970) Congenital abnormalities and anticonvulsant drugs. Proc. roy. Soc. Med., 63, 48-49

Mercier-Parot, L. & Tuchmann-Duplessis, H. (1974) The dysmorphogenic potential of phenytoin: experimental observations. Drugs, 8, 340-353

Millar, J.H.D. & Nevin, N.C. (1973) Congenital malformations and anticon-vulsant drugs. Lancet, i, 328

Mirkin, B.L. (1971) Diphenylhydantoin: placental transport, fetal localization, neonatal metabolism, and possible teratogenic effects. J. Pediat., 78, 329-337

Monson, R.R., Rosenberg, L., Hartz, S.C., Shapiro, S., Heinonen, O.P. & Slone, D. (1973) Diphenylhydantoin and selected congenital malfor-mations. New Engl. J. Med., 289, 1049-1052

Montgomery, M.R., Holtzman, J.L., Leute, R.K., Dewees, J.S. & Bolz, G. (1975) Determination of diphenylhydantoin in human serum by spin immunoassay. Clin. Chem., 21, 221-226

Morris, J.E., Price, J.M., Lalich, J.J. & Stein, R.J. (1969) The carcinogenic activity of some 5-nitrofuran derivatives in the rat.
Cancer Res., 29, 2145-2156

Morrison, L.D. & O'Donnell, C.M. (1974) Determination of diphenylhydantoin
by phosphorescence spectrometry. Analyt. Chem., 46, 1119-1120

Muñiz, F., Houston, E., Schneider, R. & Nusyowitz, M. (1969) Chromosomal
effects of diphenylhydantoins. Clin. Res., 17, 28

National Formulary Board (1970) National Formulary XIII, Washington DC,
American Pharmaceutical Association, pp. 258-259

Neuhäuser, G., Schwanitz, G. & Rott, H-D. (1970) Zur Frage mutagener und
teratogener Wirkung von Antikonvulsiva. Fortschr. Med., 88, 819-820

Niswander, J.D. & Wertelecki, W. (1973) Congenital malformation among
offspring of epileptic women. Lancet, i, 1062

Noach, E.L., Woodbury, D.M. & Goodman, L.S. (1958) Studies on the absorption, distribution, fate and excretion of $4-C^{14}$-labeled diphenylhydantoin. J. Pharmacol. exp. Ther., 122, 301-314

Pecci, J. & Giovanniello, T.J. (1975) Gas chromatographic studies of
phenobarbital and diphenylhydantoin after flash-heater alkylation.
J. Chromat., 109, 163-167

Pendergrass, T.W. & Hanson, J.W. (1976) Fetal hydantoin syndrome and
neuroblastoma. Lancet, ii, 150

Peraino, C., Fry, R.J.M., Staffeldt, E. & Christopher, J.P. (1975)
Comparative enhancing effects of phenobarbital, amobarbital, diphenylhydantoin and dichlorodiphenyltrichloroethane on 2-acetylaminofluorene-
induced hepatic tumorigenesis in the rat. Cancer Res., 35, 2884-2890

Pettifor, J.M. & Benson, R. (1975) Congenital malformations associated
with the administration of oral anticoagulants during pregnancy.
J. Pediat., 86, 459-462

Pippenger, C.E., Scott, J.E. & Gillen, H.W. (1969) Thin-layer chromatography
of anticonvulsant drugs. Clin. Chem., 15, 255-260

Prelini, R. & Gerosa, A.Z. (1975) Applicazione della densitometria
all'analisi routinaria di specialita farmaceutiche. Boll. Chim. Farm.,
114, 355-360

Rausing, A. & Trell, E. (1971) Malignant lymphogranulomatosis and anticonvulsant therapy. Acta med. scand., 189, 131-136

Roman, I.C. & Caratzali, A. (1971) Effects of anticonvulsant drugs on
chromosomes. Brit. med. J., iv, 234

Saitoh, Y., Nishihara, K., Nakagawa, F. & Suzuki, T. (1973) Improved
    microdetermination for diphenylhydantoin in blood by UV spectrophoto-
    metry. J. pharm. Sci., 62, 206-210

Saltzstein, S.L. & Ackerman, L.V. (1959) Lymphadenopathy induced by anti-
    convulsant drugs and mimicking clinically and pathologically malignant
    lymphomas. Cancer, 12, 164-182

Sherman, S. & Roizen, N. (1976) Fetal hydantoin syndrome and neuroblastoma.
    Lancet, ii, 517

Shoeman, D.W., Kauffman, R.E., Azarnoff, D.L. & Boulos, B.M. (1972)
    Placental transfer of diphenylhydantoin in the goat. Biochem. Pharmacol.,
    21, 1237-1243

Smith, E. (1966) Hydantoin. In: Kirk, R.E. & Othmer, D.F., eds,
    Encyclopedia of Chemical Technology, 2nd ed., Vol. 11, New York, John
    Wiley and Sons, p. 156

Sorrell, T.C. & Forbes, I.J. (1975) Phenytoin sensitivity in a case of
    phenytoin-associated Hodgkin's disease. Austr. N.Z. J. Med., 5, 144-147

South, J. (1972) Teratogenic effect of anticonvulsants. Lancet, ii, 1154

Speidel, B.D. & Meadow, S.R. (1972) Maternal epilepsy and abnormalities of
    the fetus and newborn. Lancet, ii, 839-843

Stecher, P.G., ed. (1968) The Merck Index, 8th ed., Rahway, NJ, Merck &
    Co., p. 388

Steinberg, A.D., Allen, P.M. & Jeffay, H. (1973) Distribution and metabolism
    of diphenylhydantoin in oral and nonoral tissues of ferrets.
    J. dent. Res., 52, 267-270

Stenchever, M.A. & Jarvis, J.A. (1971) Diphenylhydantoin: effect on
    the chromosomes of human leukocytes. Amer. J. Obstet. Gynec., 109,
    961-962

Stevens, M.W. & Harbison, R.D. (1974) Placental transfer of diphenyl-
    hydantoin: effects of species, gestational age, and route of
    administration. Teratology, 9, 317-326

Sullivan, F.M. & McElhatton, P.R. (1975) Teratogenic activity of the anti-
    epileptic drugs phenobarbital, phenytoin, and primidone in mice.
    Toxicol. appl. Pharmacol., 34, 271-282

Swinyard, E.A. (1975) Antiepileptics. In: Osol, A. et al., eds,
    Remington's Pharmaceutical Sciences, 15th ed., Easton, Pa, Mack,
    p. 1017-1018

Tashima, C.K. & de los Santos, R. (1974) Lymphoma and anticonvulsive therapy.
    J. Amer. med. Ass., 228, 286-287

Thompson, R.M., Beghin, J., Fife, W.K. & Gerber, N. (1976) 5,5-Bis(4-hydroxyphenyl)hydantoin, a minor metabolite of diphenylhydantoin (dilantin) in the rat and human. Drug Metab. Disposition, 4, 349-356

US International Trade Commission (1976a) Synthetic Organic Chemicals, US Production and Sales, 1974, USITC Publication 776, Washington DC, US Government Printing Office, p. 106

US International Trade Commission (1976b) Imports of Benzenoid Chemicals and Products, 1974, USITC Publication 762, Washington DC, US Government Printing Office, p. 83

US Pharmacopeial Convention, Inc. (1975) The US Pharmacopeia, 19th rev., Rockville, Md, pp. 379-381

US Tariff Commission (1939) Synthetic Organic Chemicals, US Production and Sales, 1938, Report No. 136, Second Series, Washington DC, US Government Printing Office, p. 36

US Tariff Commission (1948) Synthetic Organic Chemicals, US Production and Sales, 1946, Report No. 159, Second Series, Washington DC, US Government Printing Office, p. 103

US Tariff Commission (1973) Imports of Benzenoid Chemicals and Products, 1972, TC Publication 601, Washington DC, US Government Printing Office, p. 85

US Tariff Commission (1974) Imports of Benzenoid Chemicals and Products, 1973, TC Publication 688, Washington DC, US Government Printing Office, p. 81

Waddell, W.J. & Mirkin, B.L. (1972) Distribution and metabolism of diphenyl-hydantoin-^{14}C in fetal and maternal tissues of the pregnant mouse. Biochem. Pharmacol., 21, 547-552

Watson, J.D. & Spellacy, W.N. (1971) Neonatal effects of maternal treatment with the anticonvulsant drug diphenylhydantoin. Obstet. Gynec., 37, 881-885

Weast, R.C., ed. (1975) CRC Handbook of Chemistry and Physics, 56th ed., Cleveland, Ohio, Chemical Rubber Co., p. C-336

Wildhack, R. (1973) Leukämie nach Hydantoin-Behandlung. Münch. med. Wschr., 115, 1275-1279

Wilson, J.G. (1973) Present status of drugs as teratogens in man. Teratology, 7, 3-16

PRONETALOL HYDROCHLORIDE

1. Chemical and Physical Data

1.1 Synonyms and trade names

Chem. Abstr. Reg. Serial No.: 51-02-5

Chem. Abstr. Name: α-{[(1-Methylethyl)amino]methyl}-2-naphthalene-methanol, hydrochloride

Alderlin hydrochloride; α-[(isopropylamino)methyl]-2-naphthalene-methanol, hydrochloride; 2-isopropylamino-1-(2-naphthyl)ethanol hydrochloride; naphthylisoproterenol hydrochloride; pronethalol hydrochloride

ICI 38174; Inetol; Nethalide hydrochloride

1.2 Chemical formula and molecular weight

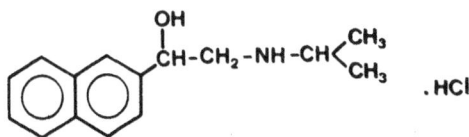

$C_{15}H_{19}NO \cdot HCl$ Mol. wt: 265.8

1.3 Chemical and physical properties of the pure substance

From Stecher (1968)

(a) Description: Crystals

(b) Melting-point: $184^{\circ}C$

1.4 Technical products and impurities

No data were available to the Working Group.

2. Production, Use, Occurrence and Analysis

For important background information on this section, see preamble, p. 15.

2.1 Production and use

(a) Production

A method of synthesizing the free base, pronetalol, by the reduction of 2-naphthacyl bromide with sodium borohydride, followed by reaction with isopropylamine, was patented in the UK in 1962 by Stephenson (Stecher, 1968).

No evidence was found that pronetalol hydrochloride has been produced commercially in the US or Japan. It has been produced by one company in Europe in the past but is no longer available.

(b) Use

Pronetalol hydrochloride is the salt of pronetalol, a potent β-adrenergic blocking agent with little sympathomimetic activity. It was withdrawn from clinical use prior to 1970 (Grollman & Grollman, 1970) because it was found to produce tumours in mice after prolonged administration (Howe *et al.*, 1968).

2.2 Occurrence

Pronetalol hydrochloride is not known to occur in nature.

2.3 Analysis

Several quantitative analytical methods, including thin-layer and gas chromatography, have been developed to determine the free base, pronetalol (Cerri, 1970).

A sensitive assay for β-adrenergic blocking drugs, including pronetalol, in biological fluids is based on the use of gas chromatography with electron-capture detection of the trifluoroacetyl derivatives. The limit of detection is in the order of 0.1 ng/ml (Walle, 1974).

3. Biological Data Relevant to the Evaluation
of Carcinogenic Risk to Man

3.1 Carcinogenicity and related studies in animals

Oral administration

Mouse: In an inadequately reported study, doses of up to 200 mg/kg bw produced lymphomas in various organs (Paget, 1963).

Groups of 25 male and 25 female mice (strain unspecified) were fed pronetalol HCl in the diet at concentrations of 0.2, 0.1, 0.05 and 0% for up to 454 days, at which time the experiment was terminated. Four thymic tumours occurred after 141, 240, 358 and 353 days in females fed a diet containing 0.1%. Three thymic tumours occurred in males fed 0.1% in the diet after 115, 329 and 450 days. Among mice fed 0.2%, 1 male and 2 females developed thymic tumours after 283, 171 and 257 days, respectively. Among mice fed 0.05%, no males and 3 females developed thymic tumours after 172, 220 and 428 days, respectively; one thymic tumour was observed in control males after 338 days (Howe, 1965).

Rat: In an adequately reported study, no tumours occurred in rats treated with doses up to 200 mg/kg bw for 2 years (Paget, 1963).

3.2 Other relevant biological data

(a) Experimental systems

The i.v. LD_{50} of pronetalol HCl in mice is about 46 mg/kg bw and the oral LD_{50} about 550 mg/kg bw (Black et $al.$, 1965).

Pronetalol HCl is absorbed rapidly from the intestine of anaesthetized dogs. In conscious dogs peak blood levels were reached about one hour after oral administration. The highest average tissue concentrations were found in the spleen, followed by kidney, brain, heart and uterus (Black & Stephenson, 1962).

Five metabolites of the drug have been identified in the urine of various species. Four of these, 2-amino-1-(2-naphthyl)ethanol, 2-naphthyl-glycolic acid, 2-naphthylglyoxylic acid and 2-naphthoic acid, are formed by degradation of the isopropylaminoethanol side-chain. The fifth, the 7-hydroxy analogue, is present partly in the free form but predominantly as its glucuronide. In mice, rats, guinea-pigs, rabbits, dogs, cats and monkeys, the differences in the major metabolites are of a quantitative rather than of a qualitative character. In most of the hitherto tested species, ring hydroxylation and conjugation is the major pathway; in guinea-pigs, side-chain oxidation is more frequent than ring hydroxylation and conjugation (Bond & Howe, 1967).

A dihydrodiol metabolite and the glycol, 1-(2-naphthyl)ethane-1,2-diol, were identified in the urine of rats, while 4 phenolic metabolites, a dihydrodiol and the glycol were detected in mouse urine. The major monohydroxylated metabolite excreted by mice was the 7-hydroxy analogue of the drug. In guinea-pig urine the glycol was the major metabolite (Stillwell & Horning, 1974).

(b) Man

In three patients treated orally with 200 mg ^{14}C-pronetalol HCl, almost all of the radioactivity was recovered from the urine within 72 hours. The excreted metabolites were similar to those found in experimental animals (Bond & Howe, 1967).

3.3 Case reports and epidemiological studies

No data were available to the Working Group.

4. Comments on Data Reported and Evaluation[1]

4.1 Animal data

Pronetalol hydrochloride is carcinogenic in mice following its oral administration: it produced thymic lymphomas.

4.2 Human data

No case reports or epidemiological studies were available to the Working Group.

---

[1]See also the section 'Animal Data in Relation to the Evaluation of Risk to Man' in the introduction to this volume, p. 13.

5. References

Black, J.W. & Stephenson, J.S. (1962) Pharmacology of a new adrenergic beta-receptor-blocking compound (nethalide). Lancet, ii, 311-314

Black, J.W., Duncan, W.A.M. & Shanks, R.G. (1965) Comparison of some properties of pronethalol and propranolol. Brit. J. Pharmacol., 25, 577-591

Bond, P.A. & Howe, R. (1967) The metabolism of pronethalol. Biochem. Pharmacol., 16, 1261-1280

Cerri, O. (1970) Determination of β-blocking drugs. Boll. Chim. Farm., 109, 338-343

Grollman, A. & Grollman, E.F. (1970) Pharmacology and Therapeutics, 7th ed., Philadelphia, Lea & Febiger, p. 311

Howe, R. (1965) Carcinogenicity of 'alderlin' (pronethalol) in mice. Nature (Lond.), 207, 594-595

Howe, R., Crowther, A.F., Stephenson, J.S., Rao, B.S. & Smith, L.H. (1968) β-Adrenergic blocking agents. I. Pronethalol and related N-alkyl and N-aralkyl derivatives of 2-amino-1-(2-naphthyl)ethanol. J. med. Chem., 11, 1000-1008

Paget, G.E. (1963) Carcinogenic action of pronethalol. Brit. med. J., iv, 1266-1267

Stecher, P.G., ed. (1968) The Merck Index, 8th ed., Rahway, NJ, Merck & Co., p. 871

Stillwell, W.G. & Horning, M.G. (1974) Metabolism of pronethalol in the rat, the guinea pig and the mouse. Res. Commun. chem. Path. Pharmacol., 9, 601-619

Walle, T. (1974) GLC determination of propranolol, other β-blocking drugs, and metabolites in biological fluids and tissues. J. pharm. Sci., 63, 1885-1891

PYRIMETHAMINE

1. Chemical and Physical Data

1.1 Synonyms and trade names

Chem. Abstr. Reg. Serial No.: 58-14-0

Chem. Abstr. Name: 5-(4-Chlorophenyl)-6-ethyl-2,4-pyrimidinediamine

5-(4'-Chlorophenyl)-2,4-diamino-6-ethylpyrimidine; 2,4-diamino-5-(4-chlorophenyl)-6-ethylpyrimidine; 2,4-diamino-5-(*para*-chlorophenyl)-6-ethylpyrimidine; pyremethamine

BW 50-63; Chloridin; Chloridine; Daraclor; Darapram; Daraprim; Daraprime; Diaminopyritamin; Erbaprelina; Erboprelina; Fansidar; Malocide; Maloprim; NSC 3061; Pirimecidan; 4753 R.P.; Tindurin

1.2 Chemical formula and molecular weight

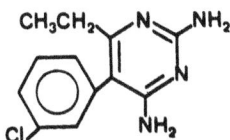

$C_{12}H_{13}ClN_4$ Mol. wt: 248.7

1.3 Chemical and physical properties of the pure substance

From Stecher (1968), unless otherwise specified

(a) Description: Crystals

(b) Melting-point: 238-242°C (US Pharmacopeial Convention, Inc., 1975)

(c) Solubility: Practically insoluble in water; very sparingly soluble in propylene glycol at 70°C and in dimethylacetamide at 70°C; slightly soluble in ethanol (0.9 g/100 ml) and in dilute hydrochloric acid (0.5 g/100 ml); soluble in boiling ethanol (2.5 g/100 ml)

1.4 Technical products and impurities

Various national and international pharmacopoeias give specifications for the purity of pyrimethamine in pharmaceutical products. For example, pyrimethamine is available in the US as a USP grade containing 99-101% active ingredient on a dried basis and as 25 mg tablets containing 93-107% of the stated amount (US Pharmacopeial Convention, Inc., 1975).

In the UK, pyrimethamine is available on a dried basis containing 99-101% of the active ingredient and as 25 mg tablets containing 92.5-107.5% of the stated amount (British Pharmacopoeia Commission, 1973). Combinations of pyrimethamine with other antimalarial drugs, e.g., chloroquine, are available in some countries.

2. Production, Use, Occurrence and Analysis

For important background information on this section, see preamble, p. 15.

2.1 Production and use

(a) Production

A method of synthesizing pyrimethamine was first patented in the US in 1951 (Hitchings *et al.*, 1951). Pyrimethamine can also be prepared by the condensation of ethyl propionate with *para*-chlorophenylacetonitrile in the presence of sodium methylate, to give α-propionyl-*para*-chlorophenylaceto-nitrile, which is then reacted with isoamyl alcohol to produce a hemiacetal. This is dehydrated to α-(*para*-chlorophenyl)-β-ethyl-β-isoamyloxyacrylo-nitrile, which is reacted with guanidine to yield pyrimethamine (Harvey, 1975).

Commercial production of pyrimethamine in the US was first reported in 1953 (US Tariff Commission, 1954); only one US company reported production in 1974 (see preamble, p. 15) (US International Trade Commission, 1976).

It has been produced in Japan since 1967, and production in 1975 was reported to be 7500 kg; 4500 kg of this were exported to south-east Asia.

Annual production of pyrimethamine in the UK is estimated to be in the range of 1-100 thousand kg.

(b) Use

Pyrimethamine is used as an antimalarial agent in human medicine. It is active against asexual blood forms in all types of malaria, producing clinical cure in all and radical cure in most cases of *Plasmodium falciparum* infection. Its action is, however, slow, and it is not, therefore, recommended for treatment of acute attacks. Pyrimethamine is a powerful suppressive agent; suppressive cure is achieved against P. *falciparum* infection and sometimes against P. *vivax* (Covell *et al.*, 1955). It is a member of a group of dihydrofolate reductase inhibitors which bind selectively to the essential enzyme of the malaria parasite, dihydrofolate reductase. Folic acid antagonism may arise with high dosages but can be prevented by concomitant administration of folinic acid (WHO, 1973).

Combinations of pyrimethamine with other drugs, such as chloroquine, quinine, sulphadoxine, sulphafurazole and sulphadiazine have been used against chloroquine-resistant falciparum malaria (WHO, 1973).

Pyrimethamine may also be used to treat toxoplasmosis, in conjunction with sulphonamide drugs such as sulphadiazine or triplesulpha (Kastrup, 1975). When used for the prophylactic treatment of toxoplasmosis in pregnancy, several courses of treatment of 25 mg twice a day are given from the 9th to the 40th week of pregnancy (Mashkovski, 1972).

Pyrimethamine has also been reported to be useful as an immunosuppressive agent (Harvey, 1975).

Use of pyrimethamine as an antimalarial agent in veterinary medicine has also been reported (Stecher, 1968). In Japan, pyrimethamine is added to domestic livestock animal feed to prevent and to suppress malarial attacks and toxoplasmosis.

2.2 Occurrence

Pyrimethamine is not known to occur in nature.

2.3 Analysis

Methods of assay for pyrimethamine that meet regulatory requirements for pharmaceutical products include non-aqueous titration and UV spectro-photometry.

Its determination in body fluids and tissues down to levels of 0.01 µg/ml can be accomplished by thin-layer chromatographic separation and UV absorption measurements on the thin-layer chromatographic plates (DeAngelis *et al.*, 1975). A similar technique, using fluorimetry, has been employed for its detection in urine, with a limit of detection of 0.1 mg/ml (Jones & King, 1968).

Pyrimethamine has been determined in animal feed by gas chromatography with electron capture detection (Royere *et al.*, 1972). Gas chromatography with both electron capture and mass spectrometry detection have been used for its determination in tissues, with a limit of detection of 0.1 mg/kg (Cala *et al.*, 1972).

It can be determined in pharmaceutical products by nuclear magnetic resonance spectroscopy (Girgis & Askam, 1974).

3. Biological Data Relevant to the Evaluation of Carcinogenic Risk to Man

3.1 Carcinogenicity and related studies in animals

Intraperitoneal administration

Mouse: In a large-scale screening study, groups of 10 male and 10 female A/He mice, 6-8 weeks old, received 5 i.p. injections over 8 weeks of pyrimethamine dissolved in 0.1 ml redistilled tricaprylin (total doses pyrimethamine, 0.125, 0.062 and 0.025 g/kg bw). Animals were killed 24 weeks after the first injection; the numbers of survivors were 9/20, 9/20 and 18/20, respectively. Control groups received 24 i.p. injections of 0.1 ml tricaprylin or were untreated; the numbers of survivors of both sexes were 154/160 and 94/100, respectively. Urethane-treated animals served as positive controls. The number of lung tumours per mouse in animals of both sexes treated with the highest dose was 0.78, which was

236

significantly higher [P<0.05] than that in untreated (0.22 in males, 0.17 in females) or vehicle-treated (0.24 in males, 0.20 in females) controls. At lower doses the increase in the number of lung tumours per mouse was not statistically significant. The numbers of mice with lung tumours (calculated on the basis of survivors of both sexes) were 5/9 (56%), 4/9 (44%) and 4/18 (22%) in the treated groups, respectively. In control groups, the results, expressed as a percentage of tumour incidence, were: 22% in males and 17% in females (untreated group) and 28% in males and 20% in females (tricaprylin-treated group). The positive control group treated with urethane had a 100% tumour incidence (Stoner et al., 1973).

3.2 Other relevant biological data

(a) Experimental systems

In rats, daily oral doses in the diet of approximately 190 mg/kg bw were lethal within 142 days. In rhesus monkeys, daily doses of 5 mg/kg bw were almost uniformly fatal within 9-18 days: 1/4 animals died within 36 days after daily doses of 2.5 mg/kg bw. Bone-marrow and renal toxicity were observed in both species (Schmidt et al., 1953).

In rhesus monkeys, ^{14}C-labelled pyrimethamine administered orally, intravenously or intramuscularly, is completely but slowly absorbed from the gastrointestinal tract and undergoes metabolism; 82-84.5% of the radioactivity was found in the urine and 3.5-5.2% in the faeces (Rollo, 1975; Smith & Schmidt, 1963).

Doses of 25-50 mg/kg administered to rats on the 9-13th day of pregnancy induced malformations in the embryo skeletons (Akimova, 1972; Kotin & Repin, 1973). Injection of 0.1-1.5 mg into the yolk sac before or up to 4 days after commencing incubation induced a high incidence of malformations in chick embryos (Stanzhevskaya, 1966).

Barilyak & Kharchenko (1973) found that concentrations of 1.5×10^{-4} g/ml in the feed caused a 3-4 fold increase in the number of X-linked recessive lethals in Drosophila melanogaster. Chromosome abnormalities have been observed in mouse bone-marrow cells (Matveeva et al., 1973) and in blastomers from pregnant rats (Dyban & Udalova, 1967) following treatment with pyrimethamine in vivo.

(b) Man

Following administration of single oral doses of 100 mg pyrimethamine
to human subjects, the average concentration in the serum fell slowly,
reaching 0.12 mg/l 9 days after dosing. Urinary excretion, which accounted
for 20-30% of the drug administered, continued for at least 30 days before
falling below detectable limits (Smith & Ihrig, 1959).

Pyrimethamine crosses the placental barrier and is also excreted in
the mother's milk (Rollo, 1975; Sadoff, 1972).

Chromosome abnormalities were observed in metaphases of bone-marrow
cells examined in 3 of 5 patients receiving total doses of 200-300 mg
pyrimethamine (Bottura & Coutinho, 1965). Chromosome abnormalities were
observed *in vitro* in human peripheral lymphocytes treated with 2.5 x 10^{-5}
g/ml (Barilyak & Kharchenko, 1973).

3.3 Case reports and epidemiological studies

It has been suggested (Sadoff, 1972) that pyrimethamine might be
incriminated in the etiology of Burkitt's lymphoma, since the drug was
introduced in tropical Africa for the suppression and treatment of malaria
in 1949, and the first cases of Burkitt's lymphoma were reported in the
area 4 years later. However, available evidence does not support the
hypothesis that Burkitt's lymphoma is a 'new disease' or that the children
affected by this malignancy, or their mothers, were treated with the drug
(Hutt & Burkitt, 1973; Williams, 1973). An apparent connection exists,
however, between malarial infection and cancer in children in Africa (see
'General Remarks on the Substances Considered', pp. 24-25).

4. Comments on Data Reported and Evaluation[1]

4.1 Animal data

In the only study available, pyrimethamine produced a significant
increase in the number of lung tumours per mouse when it was given intra-

----

[1]See also the section 'Animal Data in Relation to the Evaluation of
Risk to Man' in the introduction to this volume, p. 13.

peritoneally at high doses.   This limited evidence of carcinogenicity awaits confirmation[1].

4.2 Human data

No case reports or epidemiological studies were available to the Working Group.

---

[1]The Working Group was also aware of ongoing carcinogenicity tests in mice and rats (IARC, 1976).

5. References

Akimova, I.M. (1972) Anomalies in the development of the rat embryo skeleton after chloridine (pyrimethamine). Arkh. Anat. Gistol. Embriol., 62, 77-88

Barilyak, I.R. & Kharchenko, T.I. (1973) Investigation of the mutagenic activity of some drugs. Tsitol. Genet., 7, 455-458

Bottura, C. & Coutinho, V. (1965) The effect of pyrimethamine on the human chromosomes. Rev. Brasil. Biol., 25, 145-147

British Pharmacopoeia Commission (1973) British Pharmacopoeia, London, HMSO, p. 405

Cala, P.C., Trenner, N.R. & Buhs, R.P., Downing, G.V., Jr, Smith, J.L. & VandenHeuvel, W.J.A., III (1972) Gas chromatographic determination of pyrimethamine in tissue. J. agric. Food Chem., 20, 337-340

Covell, G., Coatney, G.R., Field, J.W. & Singh, J. (1955) Chemotherapy of malaria. Wld Hlth Org. Monogr. Ser., No. 27, pp. 51, 87

DeAngelis, R.L., Simmons, W.S. & Nichol, C.A. (1975) Quantitative thin-layer chromatography of pyrimethamine and related diaminopyrimidines in body fluids and tissues. J. Chromat., 106, 41-49

Dyban, A.P. & Udalova, L.D. (1967) A study of chromosome aberrations at the early stages of mammalian embryogenesis. I. The experiments with the effect of 2,4-diamino-5-p-chlorophenyl-6-ethyl-pyrimidine (pyrimethamine) on rats. Genetika, 4, 52-65

Girgis, P. & Askam, V. (1974) The determination of pyrimethamine by nuclear magnetic resonance spectroscopy. J. Ass. publ. Anal., 12, 55-59

Harvey, S.C. (1975) Antimicrobial drugs. In: Osol, A. *et al.*, eds, Remington's Pharmaceutical Sciences, 15th ed., Easton, Pa, Mack, p. 1159

Hitchings, G.H., Russell, P.B. & Falco, E.A. (1951) 2,4-Diamino-5-phenyl-6-alkylpyrimidines. US Patent 2,576,939, to Burroughs Wellcome and Co. (USA) Inc.

Hutt, M.S.R. & Burkitt, D.P. (1973) Aetiology of Burkitt's lymphoma. Lancet, i, 439

IARC (1976) IARC Information Bulletin on the Survey of Chemicals Being Tested for Carcinogenicity, No. 6, Lyon, p. 166

Jones, C.R. & King, L.A. (1968) Detection and fluorescent measurement of pyrimethamine in urine. Biochem. med., 2, 251-259

Kastrup, E.K., ed. (1975) *Facts and Comparisons*, St Louis, Missouri, Facts and Comparisons, Inc., p. 391

Kotin, A.M. & Repin, V.S. (1973) Effect of pyrimethamine on nucleic acid metabolism in white rat embryos. *Ontogenez*, **4**, 128-138

Mashkovski, M.D. (1972) *Drug Compounds*, Moscow, Medizina, pp. 384-385

Matveeva, V.G., Kerkis, Y.Y. & Osipova, L.I. (1973) Mutagenic effect of DDB pesticide and chloridine in bone marrow and germ cells of mice. *Genetika*, **9**, 67-76

Rollo, I.M. (1975) *Drugs used in the chemotherapy of malaria.* In: Goodman, L.S. & Gilman, A., eds, *The Pharmacological Basis of Therapeutics*, 5th ed., New York, Macmillan, pp. 1053-1058

Royere, G., Dufoir, J. & Faure, J. (1972) Dosage de la pyriméthamine dans les aliments pour animaux par chromatographie en phase gazeuse. *Analusis*, **1**, 362-364

Sadoff, L. (1972) Aetiology of Burkitt's lymphoma. *Lancet*, **ii**, 1414

Schmidt, L.H., Hughes, H.B. & Schmidt, I.G. (1953) The pharmacological properties of 2,4-diamino-5-p-chlorophenyl-6-ethylpyrimidine (Daraprim). *J. Pharmacol. exp. Ther.*, **107**, 92-130

Smith, C.C. & Ihrig, J. (1959) Persistent excretion of pyrimethamine following oral administration. *Amer. J. trop. Med. Hyg.*, **8**, 60-62

Smith, C.C. & Schmidt, L.H. (1963) Observations on the absorption of pyrimethamine from the gastrointestinal tract. *Exp. Parasitol.*, **13**, 178-185

Stanzhevskaya, T.I. (1966) The influence of chloridine on chick embryogenesis. *Bjull. eksp. Biol. Med.*, **61**, 85-88

Stecher, P.G., ed. (1968) *The Merck Index*, 8th ed., Rahway, NJ, Merck & Co., p. 892

Stoner, G.D., Shimkin, M.B., Kniazeff, A.J., Weisburger, J.H., Weisburger, E.K. & Gori, G.B. (1973) Test for carcinogenicity of food additives and chemotherapeutic agents by the pulmonary tumor response in strain A mice. *Cancer Res.*, **33**, 3069-3085

US International Trade Commission (1976) *Synthetic Organic Chemicals, US Production and Sales, 1974*, USITC Publication 776, Washington DC, US Government Printing Office, p. 101

US Pharmacopeial Convention, Inc. (1975) *The US Pharmacopeia*, 19th rev., Rockville, Md, p. 430

US Tariff Commission (1954) Synthetic Organic Chemicals, US Production and Sales, 1953, Report No. 194, Second Series, Washington DC, US Government Printing Office, p. 106

WHO (1973) Chemotherapy of malaria and resistance to antimalarials. Wld Hlth Org. techn. Rep. Ser., No. 529, pp. 16, 20-21

Williams, E.H. (1973) Aetiology of Burkitt's lymphoma. Lancet, i, 1123

SUPPLEMENTARY CORRIGENDA TO VOLUMES 1 - 12

Corrigenda covering Volumes 1 - 6 appeared in Volume 7, others appeared in Volumes 8, 10, 11 and 12.

Volume 4

p. 231   1.1   *replace* Chem. Abstr. No.: 432-88-1 *by* 542-88-1

p. 253   1.1   *replace* Chem. Abstr. No.: 1633-83-6 *by* 1120-71-4

Volume 9

p. 183   3.1(a)   *replace* 100 cm^3 *by* 0.01 ml
          2nd line

Volume 10

p. 24   Reference   *replace* (1975) *by* (1976)
         No. 32

Volume 11

p. 26   Reference   *replace* (1975) *by* (1976)
         No. 33

p. 222   References   *replace* 576-567 *by* 576-577
          last line

Volume 12

p. 22   Reference   *replace* (1975) *by* (1976)
         No. 34

p. 123   2.2   *delete from* "For information ...." *to* "see IARC (1974)."
          1st para.

CUMULATIVE INDEX TO IARC MONOGRAPHS ON THE EVALUATION
OF CARCINOGENIC RISK OF CHEMICALS TO MAN

Numbers underlined indicate volume, and numbers in italics indicate page. References to corrigenda are given in parentheses.

Acetamide	7,*197*
Acriflavinium chloride	13,*31*
Actinomycins	10,*29*
Adriamycin	10,*43*
Aflatoxins	1,*145* (corr. 7,*319*)
	(corr. 8,*349*)
	10,*51*
Aldrin	5,*25*
Amaranth	8,*41*
para-Aminoazobenzene	8,*53*
ortho-Aminoazotoluene	8,*61* (corr. 11,*295*)
4-Aminobiphenyl	1,*74* (corr. 10,*343*)
2-Amino-5-(5-nitro-2-furyl)-1,3,4-thiadiazole	7,*143*
Amitrole	7,*31*
Anaesthetics, volatile	11,*285*
Aniline	4,*27* (corr. 7,*320*)
Apholate	9,*31*
Aramite (R)	5,*39*
Arsenic and inorganic arsenic compounds	2,*48*
Arsenic (inorganic)	
Arsenic pentoxide	
Arsenic trioxide	
Calcium arsenate	
Calcium arsenite	
Potassium arsenate	
Potassium arsenite	
Sodium arsenate	
Sodium arsenite	
Asbestos	2,*17* (corr. 7,*319*)
Amosite	

Anthophyllite

Chrysotile

Crocidolite

Auramine   <u>1</u>,69   (corr. <u>7</u>,319)

Aurothioglucose   <u>13</u>,39

Azaserine   <u>10</u>,73

Aziridine   <u>9</u>,37

2-(1-Aziridinyl)ethanol   <u>9</u>,47

Aziridyl benzoquinone   <u>9</u>,51

Azobenzene   <u>8</u>,75

Benz[c]acridine   <u>3</u>,241

Benz[a]anthracene   <u>3</u>,45

Benzene   <u>7</u>,203 (corr. <u>11</u>,295)

Benzidine   <u>1</u>,80

Benzo[b]fluoranthene   <u>3</u>,69

Benzo[j]fluoranthene   <u>3</u>,82

Benzo[a]pyrene   <u>3</u>,91

Benzo[e]pyrene   <u>3</u>,137

Benzyl chloride   <u>11</u>,217 (corr. <u>13</u>,243)

Beryllium and beryllium compounds   <u>1</u>,17

    Beryl ore

    Beryllium oxide

    Beryllium phosphate

    Beryllium sulphate

BHC (technical grades)   <u>5</u>,47

Bis(1-aziridinyl)morpholinophosphine sulphide   <u>9</u>,55

Bis(2-chloroethyl)ether   <u>9</u>,117

N,N-Bis(2-chloroethyl)-2-naphthylamine   <u>4</u>,119

Bis(chloromethyl)ether   <u>4</u>,231 (corr. <u>13</u>,243)

1,4-Butanediol dimethanesulphonate   <u>4</u>,247

β-Butyrolactone   <u>11</u>,225

γ-Butyrolactone   <u>11</u>,231

Cadmium and cadmium compounds   <u>2</u>,74

                                                  <u>11</u>,39

Cadmium acetate

Cadmium carbonate

Cadmium chloride

Cadmium oxide

Cadmium powder

Cadmium sulphate

Cadmium sulphide

Cantharidin   10,*79*

Carbaryl   12,*37*

Carbon tetrachloride   1,*53*

Carmoisine   8,*83*

Chlorambucil   9,*125*

Chloramphenicol   10,*85*

Chlormadinone acetate   6,*149*

Chlorobenzilate   5,*75*

Chloroform   1,*61*

Chloromethyl methyl ether   4,*239*

Chloropropham   12,*55*

Chloroquine   13,*47*

Cholesterol   10,*99*

Chromium and inorganic chromium compounds   2,*100*

    Barium chromate

    Calcium chromate

    Chromic chromate

    Chromic oxide

    Chromium acetate

    Chromium carbonate

    Chromium dioxide

    Chromium phosphate

    Chromium trioxide

    Lead chromate

    Potassium chromate

    Potassium dichromate

    Sodium chromate

    Sodium dichromate

Strontium chromate

Zinc chromate hydroxide

Chrysene   3,*159*

Chrysoidine   8,*91*

C.I. Disperse Yellow 3   8,*97*

Citrus Red No. 2   8,*101*

Coumarin   10,*113*

Cycasin   1,*157* (corr. 7,*319*)

     10,*121*

Cyclochlorotine   10,*139*

Cyclophosphamide   9,*135*

Daunomycin   10,*145*

D & C Red No. 9   8,*107*

DDT and associated substances   5,*83* (corr. 7,*320*)

     DDD (TDE)

     DDE

Diacetylaminoazotoluene   8,*113*

Diallate   12,*69*

2,6-Diamino-3-(phenylazo)pyridine (hydrochloride)   8,*117*

Diazepam   13,*57*

Diazomethane   7,*223*

Dibenz[a,h]acridine   3,*247*

Dibenz[a,j]acridine   3,*254*

Dibenz[a,h]anthracene   3,*178*

7H-Dibenzo[c,g]carbazole   3,*260*

Dibenzo[h,rst]pentaphene   3,*197*

Dibenzo[a,e]pyrene   3,*201*

Dibenzo[a,h]pyrene   3,*207*

Dibenzo[a,i]pyrene   3,*215*

Dibenzo[a,l]pyrene   3,*224*

ortho-Dichlorobenzene   7,*231*

para-Dichlorobenzene   7,*231*

3,3'-Dichlorobenzidine   4,*49*

Dieldrin   5,*125*

Diepoxybutane   11,*115*

1,2-Diethylhydrazine   <u>4</u>,*153*

Diethylstilboestrol   <u>6</u>,*55*

Diethyl sulphate   <u>4</u>,*277*

Diglycidyl resorcinol ether   <u>11</u>,*125*

Dihydrosafrole   <u>1</u>,*170*

                                                                      <u>10</u>,*233*

Dimethisterone   <u>6</u>,*167*

3,3'-Dimethoxybenzidine (*o*-Dianisidine)   <u>4</u>,*41*

para-Dimethylaminoazobenzene   <u>8</u>,*125*

para-Dimethylaminobenzenediazo sodium sulphonate   <u>8</u>,*147*

trans-2[(Dimethylamino)methylimino]-5-[2-(5-nitro-
   2-furyl)vinyl]-1,3,4-oxadiazole   <u>7</u>,*147*

3,3'-Dimethylbenzidine (*o*-Tolidine)   <u>1</u>,*87*

Dimethylcarbamoyl chloride   <u>12</u>,*77*

1,1-Dimethylhydrazine   <u>4</u>,*137*

1,2-Dimethylhydrazine   <u>4</u>,*145* (corr. <u>7</u>,*320*)

Dimethyl sulphate   <u>4</u>,*271*

Dinitrosopentamethylenetetramine   <u>11</u>,*241*

1,4-Dioxane   <u>11</u>,*247*

Disulfiram   <u>12</u>,*85*

Dithranol   <u>13</u>,*75*

Dulcin   <u>12</u>,*97*

Endrin   <u>5</u>,*157*

Epichlorohydrin   <u>11</u>,*131*

1-Epoxyethyl-3,4-epoxycyclohexane   <u>11</u>,*141*

3,4-Epoxy-6-methylcyclohexylmethyl-3,4-epoxy-
   6-methylcyclohexane carboxylate   <u>11</u>,*147*

cis-9,10-Epoxystearic acid   <u>11</u>,*153*

Ethinyloestradiol   <u>6</u>,*77*

Ethionamide   <u>13</u>,*83*

Ethylene oxide   <u>11</u>,*157*

Ethylene sulphide   <u>11</u>,*257*

Ethylenethiourea   <u>7</u>,*45*

Ethyl methanesulphonate   <u>7</u>,*245*

Ethyl selenac   <u>12</u>,*107*

Ethyl tellurac   12,*115*

Ethynodiol diacetate   6,*173*

Evans blue   8,*151*

Ferbam   12,*121* (corr. 13,*243*)

2-(2-Formylhydrazino)-4-(5-nitro-2-furyl)thiazole   7,*151* (corr. 11,*295*)

Fusarenon-X   11,*169*

Glycidaldehyde   11,*175*

Glycidyl oleate   11,*183*

Glycidyl stearate   11,*187*

Griseofulvin   10,*153*

Haematite   1,*29*

Heptachlor and its epoxide   5,*173*

Hycanthone   13,*91*

Hycanthone mesylate   13,*92*

Hydrazine   4,*127*

4-Hydroxyazobenzene   8,*157*

8-Hydroxyquinoline   13,*101*

Hydroxysenkirkine   10,*265*

Indeno[1,2,3-*cd*]pyrene   3,*229*

Iron-dextran complex   2,*161*

Iron-dextrin complex   2,*161* (corr. 7,*319*)

Iron oxide   1,*29*

Iron sorbitol-citric acid complex   2,*161*

Isatidine   10,*269*

Isonicotinic acid hydrazide   4,*159*

Isosafrole   1,*169*

                                                        10,*232*

Jacobine   10,*275*

Lasiocarpine   10,*281*

Lead salts   1,*40* (corr. 7,*319*)

                                                              (corr. 8,*349*)

   Lead acetate

   Lead arsenate

   Lead carbonate

   Lead phosphate

Lead subacetate

Ledate   12,*131*

Lindane   5,*47*

Luteoskyrin   10,*163*

Magenta   4,*57*   (corr. 7,*320*)

Maleic hydrazide   4,*173*

Maneb   12,*137*

Mannomustine (dihydrochloride)   9,*157*

Medphalan   9,*167*

Medroxyprogesterone acetate   6,*157*

Melphalan   9,*167*

Merphalan   9,*167*

Mestranol   6,*87*

Methoxychlor   5,*193*

2-Methylaziridine   9,*61*

Methylazoxymethanol acetate   1,*164*
                                                10,*131*

Methyl carbamate   12,*151*

N-Methyl-N,4-dinitrosoaniline   1,*141*

4,4'-Methylene bis(2-chloroaniline)   4,*65*

4,4'-Methylene bis(2-methylaniline)   4,*73*

4,4'-Methylenedianiline   4,*79*   (corr. 7,*320*)

Methyl methanesulphonate   7,*253*

N-Methyl-N'-nitro-N-nitrosoguanidine   4,*183*

Methyl red   8,*161*

Methyl selenac   12,*161*

Methylthiouracil   7,*53*

Metronidazole   13,*113*

Mirex   5,*203*

Mitomycin C   10,*171*

Monocrotaline   10,*291*

Monuron   12,*167*

5-(Morpholinomethyl)-3-[(5-nitrofurfurylidene)-
   amino]-2-oxazolidinone   7,*161*

Mustard gas   9,*181* (corr. 13,*243*)

1-Naphthylamine   _4_,*87* (corr. _8_,*349*)

2-Naphthylamine   _4_,*97*

Native carrageenans   _10_,*181* (corr. _11_,*295*)

Nickel and nickel compounds   _2_,*126* (corr. _7_,*319*)

    _11_,*75*

     Nickel acetate

     Nickel carbonate

     Nickel carbonyl

     Nickelocene

     Nickel oxide

     Nickel powder

     Nickel subsulphide

     Nickel sulphate

Niridazole   _13_,*123*

4-Nitrobiphenyl   _4_,*113*

5-Nitro-2-furaldehyde semicarbazone   _7_,*171*

1[(5-Nitrofurfurylidene)amino]-2-imidazolidinone   _7_,*181*

_N_-[4-(5-Nitro-2-furyl)-2-thiazolyl]acetamide   _1_,*181*

    _7_,*185*

Nitrogen mustard (hydrochloride)   _9_,*193*

Nitrogen mustard _N_-oxide (hydrochloride)   _9_,*209*

_N_-Nitrosodi-_n_-butylamine   _4_,*197*

_N_-Nitrosodiethylamine   _1_,*107* (corr. _11_,*295*)

_N_-Nitrosodimethylamine   _1_,*95*

_N_-Nitrosoethylurea   _1_,*135*

_N_-Nitrosomethylurea   _1_,*125*

_N_-Nitroso-_N_-methylurethane   _4_,*211*

Norethisterone   _6_,*179*

Norethisterone acetate   _6_,*179*

Norethynodrel   _6_,*191*

Norgestrel   _6_,*201*

Ochratoxin A   _10_,*191*

Oestradiol-17β   _6_,*99*

Oestradiol mustard   _9_,*217*

Oestriol   _6_,*117*

Oestrone   6,*123*

Oil Orange SS   8,*165*

Orange I   8,*173*

Orange G   8,*181*

Oxazepam   13,*58*

Oxymetholone   13,*131*

Oxyphenbutazone   13,*185*

Parasorbic acid   10,*199*

Patulin   10,*205*

Penicillic acid   10,*211*

Phenacetin   13,*141*

Phenicarbazide   12,*177*

Phenobarbital   13,*157*

Phenobarbital sodium   13,*159*

Phenoxybenzamine (hydrochloride)   9,*223*

Phenylbutazone   13,*183*

Phenytoin   13,*201*

Phenytoin sodium   13,*202*

Polychlorinated biphenyls   7,*261*

Ponceau MX   8,*189*

Ponceau 3R   8,*199*

Ponceau SX   8,*207*

Potassium bis(2-hydroxyethyl)dithiocarbamate   12,*183*

Progesterone   6,*135*

Pronetalol hydrochloride   13,*227*

1,3-Propane sultone   4,*253* (corr. 13,*843*)

Propham   12,*189*

β-Propiolactone   4,*259*

n-Propyl carbamate   12,*201*

Propylene oxide   11,*191*

Propylthiouracil   7,*67*

Pyrimethamine   13,*233*

Quintozene (Pentachloronitrobenzene)   5,*211*

Reserpine   10,*217*

Retrorsine   10,*303*

Riddelliine   10,*313*

Saccharated iron oxide	2,161
Safrole	1,169
	10,231
Scarlet red	8,217
Selenium and selenium compounds	9,245
Semicarbazide (hydrochloride)	12,209
Seneciphylline	10,319
Senkirkine	10,327
Sodium diethyldithiocarbamate	12,217
Soot, tars and shale oils	3,22
Sterigmatocystin	1,175
	10,245
Streptozotocin	4,221
Styrene oxide	11,201
Sudan I	8,225
Sudan II	8,233
Sudan III	8,241
Sudan brown RR	8,249
Sudan red 7B	8,253
Sunset yellow FCF	8,257
Tannic acid	10,253
Tannins	10,254
Terpene polychlorinates (Strobane[(R)])	5,219
Testosterone	6,209
Tetraethyllead	2,150
Tetramethyllead	2,150
Thioacetamide	7,77
Thiouracil	7,85
Thiourea	7,95
Thiram	12,225
Trichloroethylene	11,263
Trichlorotriethylamine hydrochloride	9,229
Triethylene glycol diglycidyl ether	11,209
Tris(aziridinyl)-*para*-benzoquinone	9,67
Tris(1-aziridinyl)phosphine oxide	9,75

Tris(1-aziridinyl)phosphine sulphide	**9**,*85*
2,4,6-Tris(1-aziridinyl)-*s*-triazine	**9**,*95*
Tris(2-methyl-1-aziridinyl)phosphine oxide	**9**,*107*
Trypan blue	**8**,*267*
Uracil mustard	**9**,*235*
Urethane	**7**,*111*
Vinyl chloride	**7**,*291*
4-Vinylcyclohexene	**11**,*277*
Yellow AB	**8**,*279*
Yellow OB	**8**,*287*
Zectran	**12**,*237*
Zineb	**12**,*245*
Ziram	**12**,*259*

www.ingramcontent.com/pod-product-compliance
Lightning Source LLC
Chambersburg PA
CBHW081808200326
41597CB00023B/4184